PAIN HEROES

Stories of Hope and Recovery

Alison Sim

ISBN: 978-0-6483250-0-0 (print)
ISBN: 978-0-6483250-1-7 (ebook)

INTRODUCTION

Pain is experienced by everyone at some point in their life. Some people experience pain that hangs around far longer than it should. This books tells the stories of people who have experienced persistent pain and recovered from it. It also gives some practical, evidence based advice on how to embrace what modern science tells us about pain in order to recover. No quick fixes or magic silver bullets, just sensible advice that is echoed by the lived experiences in the stories of the Pain Heroes.

The people in these stories have generously given their time and permission to share their story because they believe that it has value to other people who have pain. Each of these individuals have had pain that has had a significant impact on their life. It made them feel miserable, disconnected from friends and family and might have made them unable to work or look after their families. In some cases, they felt so despondent that they did not want to live any more. This is what pain can do. It can pervade every bit of a person's life, taking away the good bits and leaving behind distress, medical appointments, medication side effects, and misery. As a clinician who works with people in pain, I often find that I can look at a person who is in front of me and know that they can do really well using a modern pain science approach to getting better. An approach that understands that a person in pain is more than just the sore back, headache or persistent neck ache that they present with. One that recognises that our thoughts are important in how a condition will present itself. One that acknowledges a massive body of scientific evidence that says that movement is one of the important keys in getting better. One that focuses less on body parts that are broken or damaged and more on rehabilitation. The big problem is, for that person sitting in front of me, these messages can be really hard to hear. It can be hard to believe that getting off the merri-go-round search for a cure for their condition is possible or even necessary. I know that it will help them – but understandably, they will often find it hard to embrace. I see the skepticism in their eyes, the jaded looks that tell of multiple failed therapies and practitioners who have not believed them in the past. I want to show them the science – all of the science that can tell them that this can work for them and that this is how it works. But when I put myself in their shoes, I totally understand why they might be hesitant to embrace such an approach. Why my "trust me" appeals might fall on deaf ears.

For that person in front of me who has been through a long, expensive, frustrating and ultimately painful journey, sometimes "trust me" just does not cut it! I decided to write this book to show to people in pain that there is hope for recovery. I wanted them to see that there are people who have gone on to do really well after a long pain journey. However in the beginning they had sat there and had those exact same hesitations and doubts. I wanted to show that when they took those steps towards taking back ownership of their journey, things gradually started to improve.

In the first part of this book are the stories from eight people who were kind enough to allow me to interview them about their pain journey and their recovery. The stories, while differing in their pain presentations, have some incredibly consistent themes. Firstly, the devastation that pain brought to their life. Careers that have to be abandoned, children that are brought up by friends, financial hardship that affects whole families and associated anxiety and depression that can lead a person to feel that life is not worth living. Pain severely interferes with these people's lives. But we also see a consistent turning point in each story – one that usually involves the person learning more about what modern pain science tells us about why pain hangs around when it probably shouldn't. You will notice that once people understand some of these key messages, they feel less distressed with the presence of pain. They become more empowered to get back to doing the things that they have been avoiding and ultimately take gradual steps to do just that. Towards the end of their journey many of the people no longer identify as a person with pain anymore, others find that they still have pain but it is just not a big deal for them like it used to be. Most importantly though, they get back to life – to the things that they love that pain had taken from them.

Pain science has come a long way in the last 20 years and the information that it tells us is beginning to trickle down to our mainstream medical models. Understanding more about pain is the consistent precursor to things getting better for the people interviewed. If we could summarise three of the key points about what they learnt about pain they would be:

1. Pain is not equal to tissue damage
2. To get better, focus on function and not on pain.
3. Getting back to doing things is possible, but needs to be done very slowly and consistently

Understanding the first point really well can in itself be incredibly liberating for people. In 2004, a researcher named Lorimer Moseley published a study in the Clinical Journal of Pain whereby he emphasised these key messages from modern pain science to a group of around 30 patients with low back. On a one to one basis, he sat with each of these people for 3 hours and explained to them what we know about pain. He drew on the science that says that when we use active approaches, which are things that we can do to help ourselves like exercise, stretching and pacing, we get better compared to when we use passive interventions which are things that are done to us like massage, injections and medication. He explained that tissues in the body will heal within 3-6 months and that after healing has occurred the tissues are safe and are unlikely to become damaged further. He outlined how the nervous system changes to become more sensitive so that rather than telling that true picture of exactly what is going on in the tissues as it did at the beginning of an injury, those messages over time become slightly less accurate and will err on the side of over-exageration in order to protect what the brain perceives to be a threat – meaning that whilst the pain is real, it does not really tell a story of tissue damage. He continually emphasised that their tissues were safe and they could regain function, but that in order to regain function, a slow and steady approach was needed. He debunked the idea that what we see on our scans and x-rays will equate with how a person experiences pain – telling people about the high percentages of people who have disc bulges, osteoarthritis or degenerative changes on scans but have no pain at all.

Prior to the information session the researchers took

physical measurement and also some surveys asking about their perceptions about pain and how worried they were about the presence of pain. In the days following the three hour information session, they re-measured the physical measurements and repeated the surveys. They found that people consistently performed better on the physical testing – bending towards the floor or having their leg lifted off the bed and that they were less distressed about their pain and more confident in their bodies. The results were not enough to change a person's life immediately – they were small changes, but enough to create a foundational understanding from which that person could continue to make incremental improvements. This was compared to a control group who were exposed to different education material – about lifting, anatomy of the spine and other "old school" ideas about back pain. The control group made no change to either their physical function test or to the surveys about the distress surrounding their back pain.

Understanding more about pain can be seen as an intervention in itself – it can be a great platform from which a person can confidently begin to start getting better. It acknowledges that pain is both a physical and emotional experience and that if we don't take into account this bigger picture, we are missing some great opportunities to help people get better. In many of these instances for the people interviewed, this understanding came about after being told the information by a practitioner – some in a pain program and others in clinical practice. Other people were helped along by reading the book "Explain Pain" which was written by Lorimer Moseley (the researcher above) and David Butler. It remains in our industry as the "go to" book for chronic pain. Other resources that aim to convey similar messages are available and the details about some of these can be found at the end of the book.

The second section of the book following on from the stories is some information on the science of chronic pain. There is also guidance on how to use this information to get back to doing the things that pain has taken away.

KAREN LITZY

I had chronic neck pain for about 8 years. It started when I was about 30 years old. I woke up one morning and I couldn't get out of bed because I was in so much pain. I couldn't lift my upper body or sit up and I couldn't even call out to my room mate to ask her for help because it hurt too much. I lay there for a while and then I log rolled off the bed and fell onto the floor – it was the only way that I could get off the bed. I crawled across the floor and then when I did eventually manage to stand up, I felt like my head weighed a hundred pounds and that it was going to roll off my neck. It felt like my neck couldn't support the weight of my head. It felt really unstable and my natural instinct was to want to put a cervical collar on it to support it.

I was working as a physical therapist (physiotherapist) in New York at the time and so I started to get dressed and make my way to work. I held my neck with my hands as I walked down the four flights of stairs in my apartment. There was no way I could take the subway so I just got in a cab and when I arrived at work one of the therapists took a look at my neck for me. I had never felt pain like it before and in hindsight I probably should have gone to the emergency room for pain relief rather than going to work. I had previously had surgery on my shoulder and had many injuries as an elite gymnast in my teens and twenties but never had I experienced pain like this – it was all consuming. I couldn't get away from it because it affected my whole body and every movement.

I didn't see anyone else for it. It got a little better over the week. I regained more mobility and was able to function a bit better but the pain wasn't really going away. This was the start of the long journey with this neck pain for me. Over the next few years, there would be times when the pain would be less of a problem and times when it would be extremely painful, but it never went away. I saw it as a huge interruption to my life and it really upset me.

The pain always came on after episodes in the night. I would roll over and feel a pop and then extreme pain would follow. Sometimes I would have to take a day off work. It was really distressing and I still thought that it was a pinched nerve or a pulled muscle.

I finally went to see a doctor for it many months down the track and had an MRI scan which showed 4 or 5 herniated discs in my neck. Not long after that I was sent to a pain management doctor. My symptoms had worsened so that I was having numbness, tingling and weakness into both my hands. I was having trouble holding a pen and gripping things, especially in the mornings was a problem. My pain levels never really dropped below a five out of ten and sometimes they were very high. I was still managing to get to work nearly all of the time though.

The pain management doctor discovered some weaknesses in my left hand that I hadn't really been aware of. It was really upsetting because it was a movement I wouldn't normally perform in isolation but it had a lot of meaning because I knew that it meant that there was nerve involvement and I viewed it as being a big deal. I had an epidural in my neck not long after that evaluation, which was about a year after the onset of the pain, and almost immediately after the procedure I was able to do those specific movements. This was reassuring to me because in my interpretation of things, there had been some pressure around the nerves that were causing some inflammation, the epidural had reduced that inflammation and things should be good from here. Unfortunately though, the pain didn't subside.

I rarely missed days of work because I am a determined worker bee. I would soldier on and work even if my pain levels were high. In hindsight I can see that I was really fearful of moving my neck and doing anything that I though would aggravate it. I was particularly fearful around sleep because that was often when it would kick off – with that pop after a certain movement in bed.

About a year later following that first epidural the pain worsened and some of the muscle symptoms had started to come back again – I had some tremors in my forearm when my wrist was in particular positions. The episodes of extreme pain were also becoming more common and I went for two more epidurals about 3 months apart. Again, they helped a little but the pain wasn't getting much better.

I saw another pain management doctor who was doing nasopalatine treatment where they dipped these very long cotton tips into a mixture of narcotic solutions and other medications and would put them up both your nostrils. You would sit there with these big long q-tips up your nose for an hour, next to all these other people sitting in lounge chairs in the clinic also with q-tips up their nose. They were all a lot older than me. I was in my early 30s. I would go there when I was in really acute pain. I'd be crying and walking like the tin man. I felt really supported by that clinic and the staff and treatment actually really helped my pain levels. I would go four days in a row and then I would find that my pain levels would drop and I would be good for a couple of weeks. Then it would come back again and I would repeat the process.

The paradoxical thing is that throughout the entire time with my neck pain, I continued to play softball every Saturday, often double headers. I was the pitcher. It was just a given that I was going to play – I never questioned that I would stop that because I loved it. I never missed a game because of my neck pain. Now that I look at it through a biopsychosocial or bigger picture lens, I can see that it gave me so much joy to be playing that it didn't really make the pain worse. I loved hanging out with my team mates, I loved to play – I was good at it and so it was obviously a really positive thing for me to keep doing. I would be sore the next day but I would ice it down, and I didn't tend to focus on the soreness much. Again in hindsight, the physicality of being able to actually perform those movements was completely at odds with the view that I had of myself and my neck being fragile.

During the middle of this period of time I was taking an education course with a very good friend of mine. During the course she was doing some gentle work on my neck – really just holding it in her hands and I had some sort of reaction to the treatment. I went completely cold and started shaking and crying. I couldn't stop and we needed to leave the course and go home. I was really not doing well all that afternoon. My friend wouldn't leave me at my apartment alone until my flatmate came home. I was so worried that I rang a doctor friend to ask if I should go to the emergency room. In hindsight I think I might have had a panic attack. I hadn't been worried about people touching my neck prior to that but I have had a lot of trouble with it since. I really don't like people touching me at all, not even having a pedicure or massage.

I was really identifying as being a person with neck pain. All of my Christmas presents at the time were things like heat pads and special pillows, rolling suitcases so that I didn't have to carry anything. Also by this time I had completely stopped carrying things because I was worried it would hurt my neck. I would have groceries delivered, I would only ever carry a small purse with necessities. I would never lift things over my head. I had stopped running and doing group exercises. I was completely avoiding any pain because I thought that it was damaging me and would make the pain worse.

Sleeping was a big deal at this time because I was really fearful that the pain was going to start. I worried about it happening and so I didn't sleep well which I have no doubt made my pain worse. I got so worried about sleep that I made myself a device that held my head in one position so that the pop wouldn't happen overnight and start a flare up of the pain. I had to take this thing with me wherever I went – it was like my safety blanket.

I was in my 30s and felt like my life was on hold. Many of my friends were getting married and having kids and I felt like I couldn't have any of that because I would be such a burden to a partner. I stopped hanging out with all of those friends because it just reminded me of what I didn't have and what I couldn't ever see myself having. Because why would someone want to be with me when I couldn't get out of bed some days? Why would they choose me when they could be with someone more physically able?

About 5 years ago, so maybe 7 years into this pain, a friend of mine suggested that I come down to Washington DC to go to an education event for physical therapists where this Australian physiotherapist David Butler was speaking. She thought that I might like his work and at the time I had started the podcast so I thought that he might be good to interview. I reached out to his people to see if I could organise to interview him and in the meantime I started to read everything that he had written, including Explain Pain. It made a bit of sense to me – I hadn't considered pain like that before as I had a very biomedical approach to pain from my training.

I saw him speak and as I sat there and listened I had tears rolling down my face because everything that he said was everything that I had been experiencing. It was my first exposure to psychosocial concepts in pain. Everything that he was saying was my life. I went up to speak with him afterwards and he said that he unfortunately didn't have time to do the interview right then and there. Instead he suggested that he meet with me in New York as that was where he was heading with his wife on the next part of their vacation. He came to the office building that I worked at in New York which was incredibly gracious and kind of him. I spoke with him for two whole hours and part of it was him talking with me about my own pain.

He asked me in that interview what I did for exercise and I told him that I wasn't really doing anything. He asked me why not and I said because I was worried it was going to hurt my neck. He asked me what about running was actually going to hurt my neck. I couldn't really answer him because I guess I knew that running wasn't something that would physically damage my neck.

He gave me some homework to do which was essential graded exposure. He would get me to walk to the grocery store and get a bag of chips and a loaf of bread and carry it home. Then each time I went I had to get a few more things to put in the bag. This went on for a few months and I started to realise that I could carry things and that my neck was okay. Then he got me to go to the gym and do just a few things or a few different machines. I gradually built that up to a point where I could go and do a reasonable workout at the gym without upsetting my neck. Once I had understood more about what pain was by listening to his lectures, reading all of the books and articles that he and Lorimer Moseley had published, my pain dropped by about 80% in three months. It was really powerful understanding that my neck was safe and that pain didn't equate to damage. I started having some mornings where I would wake up without pain. This was something that never happened – I had pain every morning normally.

I kept making progress. David kept checking in on

me to make sure I was continuing to progress my exercise and that I was staying on track. It took about about another two months but gradually my pain went away. I would have occasional flare ups of pain but when it happened I would just say to myself – you are ok, you are ok, and then I would go to the gym. I have much better coping strategies now and I know that if it did come back I could cope – I wouldn't freak out – I'd just adjust my behavior for a short while and then get back to it.

I'm going really well with my gym program and have started lifting some weights this year. I am working towards being able to do a handstand.

I look back on that time as such a waste of those years. I wish I hadn't freaked out so much about the pain and I wish I hadn't let it drive every facet of my life like it did.

Karen is a well known physical therapist in New York. She runs a podcast called Healthy, Wealthy and Smart which can be downloaded from podcast apps.

PETE MOORE

My story is a really common one. I had niggly back pain at times since I was a teenager and I would just take some over the counter medication and get on with life. I didn't like stretching or exercising at the time. I didn't really look after myself – didn't eat the right foods, things like that. I was a painter and decorator and I was painting a house opposite Windsor Castle – coincidentally it was the same day that Windsor Castle went up in smoke! I went home that day after work with pain and then couldn't get out of bed the next day. I had this pain down my back and it was also going down my legs. I took the over the counter medication but nothing really helped and I didn't go to work. After about a week off work and still with the pain, I went and saw the GP. He gave me some stronger pain killers – some anti-inflammatories and an opioid based medication. Still nothing really touched the pain so I went back and he organised an x-ray. I hadn't been down this route before – I was in the shit! I was scared – I was having all these tests which meant that it must be something serious. I was stuck in what i know now is the medical model – I call it being a health tourist. I was seeing physiotherapists, trying new medications, going back to the GP every two weeks. I had an MRI, x-rays and lots of medical appointments taking up my time. I tried to go back to work – I had two jobs and I was self employed at both. I was a painter/decorator and also a driving instructor. I tried to get back to the driving instructing but I couldn't sit so I found that too difficult. I couldn't be upright for long so I just didn't have much hope about going back to work.

I was really confused at this time. In hindsight I realise that I had handed all my power over to the medical model – I was expecting to just go into the doctor and that they would do something or give you something and I would be better and go on my way. I was getting all these really different and really negative messages. I was getting some physiotherapy but I had a different therapist every time – I had to keep explaining my story each time and most of the visits they would just look at the chart and then put me on a traction rack. They would give me exercises – 10 of these ones, 8 of these ones – but when I did them, I would get up to the third one and be in so much pain. I started to learn and believe that exercise equalled pain and harm. It felt like a one size fits all approach – they were seeing 3 or 4 patients at the same time and it wasn't individually tailored.

Months down the track, I was getting worse and still hadn't returned to work. I had started to work my life around my pain – mostly around my appointments. I sold my driving school car and I bought a van specifically so that if I did go out I could lie down in the back of the van. I had modified my TV so that I could see it when I was lying on the floor. I had used all my savings – by this stage I had started to see lots of other health professionals – I would try anything – massage, chiropractors, osteopaths. None of it helped. I spent about 8000 pounds on them. I was so desperate I even visited a guy to wave a crystal around my head – I was sitting there thinking "what has my life come to – why am I doing this crap and paying 40 quid for it?"

I was referred to the orthopaedic surgeons. He told me my spine was like a digestive biscuit. Of course when you hear that you think you need to be extra careful. Things were really bad by this stage. Monday, Tuesday, Wednesday, Thursday, Friday, Saturday and Sunday – They were just names of the day really – they had no meaning to me. Every day just melted into the next. I would wake up in the morning and just ask myself how much pain I was going to be in today. My day revolved around TV programs. My friends stopped catching up with me. I understand why – the pain was the centre of my universe and I was so negative. It was all I could talk about and I get why they stopped calling. No one wants to just hear all that negative stuff. They gave up on me. I don't blame them. It's boring!

I wasn't going out at all. I couldn't walk too long. There was a supermarket that was about 10 minutes away and I would hobble up there. I would look in the window and if there was a queue I would turn around and go home. I could hardly even stand in the shower – I was so de-conditioned. I hated the look of the ceilings – because I spent so much time looking at them. I was still taking the anti-inflammatories and the opioid medications – they were just taking the edge off things.

To survive financially I was on the benefit system. All in all, while I was in that system I cost the taxpayer about 350,000 pounds.

I was stuck like this from 1992 and by the end of 1993 I realised that I had to do something, I wanted to see if I could learn from other people. I was starting to get depression by this stage. I started up this back pain support group. I found a venue and did a press release – I'd never done anything like that in my life but the local newspaper was really helpful. They did a small piece in the paper and on that very first night about 70 people turned up! The hall was only set up for 30 so people had to stand. I thought I was doing the right thing but in actual fact I was actually probably just promoting doctor shopping. We had orthopedic surgeons, chiropractors, aromatherapists, osteopaths. I ran it about one every month or every two months.

During this time, someone told me about the INPUT program in London and it sounded good so I wrote to them and asked if they would send someone down to speak to the group. They said that we would have to pay for it – but I told them we didn't have any money for that sort of thing. In the end they send Amanda Williams down and she was great. She talked about pacing and lots of other things as well as the program itself. I think by this stage I had started to realise that the answer to my problems didn't lie with one more doctor or one more type of treatment. The things she was talking about reso-nated with me. That was in 1994 and I registered for the program but I still had to wait another 18 months before I could get on the program.

At this stage things were still really going down the toilet. My darkest days. The worst one was my birthday in 1994, which is also new years eve, and I had had my full quota of meds already. Some mates came around to take me out and I couldn't go because I was in too much pain. I thought about it and started talking to the big bloke in the sky. I said "If this is what my life is going to be like now, I want to get out of the cab now". I was going to take the rest of the pills that night and end it. I couldn't see straight. It was new years eve, everyone was going out but here I was again, laying down and looking at the ceiling and the crap TV. Don't ask me what made me do it, but I decided to do some stretching – I lay on my back and stretched my leg up in the doorway and it made the pain ease off a tiny bit. It came back again crazier the next day, but even with that, I realised that I had to take action. I had to keep focused on waiting for the INPUT program and maybe keep trying to help myself.

In a way, even though we weren't really finding answers, the back pain group that I was running was therapy for me. It made me learn to use a computer so that I could type things up. I had to stay in touch with everyone to make it stay together. I did up a newsletter and kept the group going. People kept saying to me, "Pete you do so much for the group" and I would think "bugger off – I'm doing it to keep myself sane and give me something to do". People would also phone me up to talk. I had quite a few phone calls from people who were really desperate and sometimes even suicidal. People would cry on the phone – I was learning how to deal with other people in pain.

In 1996 I finally got onto the program. It was a two week residential program and I loved it. I wished it had gone on longer. Even though I had been waiting for 18 months for the program, and I'd heard Amanda speak about what it was about, I still think a part of me was stuck in that model where I just went in and they did something for me to fix it. But actually what happened was that I went in there and got off my butt and did something for myself. They weren't brutal though – they did it in a nice way. It was a residential program so you stayed there for the whole time. I was moaning one day and my physiotherapist asked me what was wrong. I told her I had a bad back. She asked me what I had been diagnosed with and I told her I had degenerated discs. She said that everyone over the age of 21 has some degeneration in their discs. I knew I had to get on with it and I knew that after the program you had to be self reliant.

I wish there had been an ex-patient of the program there to tell us about how they had gone. Because there were times when we were there in the program and we would be thinking – well it's all well and good for you to be saying that – you are a health professional. Do you even know what its like to get up in the morning and be in so much pain, do know what its like to have depression, no money? To worry – what is today going to be like? How am I going to get through? Sometimes it's so hard to see that getting over that with a pain management approach is possible. People probably need to hear that this is the best thing and that it is not just for really disabled people. They need to know that there is hope but you have to start taking charge of yourself and stop being a passenger.

One of the great things that I learnt was pacing. On day one they picked us up and they kept stopping on the way there – I was thinking – can we just hurry up and get there? But it was to teach us to take regular breaks even though we didn't feel like we needed it. We did some psychology stuff – learning to challenge our thoughts. There were relaxation components – I wasn't too good at them but they were good to learn. We did some goal setting – long and short term goals. They taught us a battle plan – set a goal and then an action plan for how to get to those goals. I also had a meeting with the nurse and they suggested that I come off my meds. I was really wary of that – it was like taking my crutch away. In the back of my mind I was also concerned that if I came off all my meds, I wouldn't be eligible for benefits any more. That worried me. I still couldn't even walk properly at that time – I walked funny and knew that no one would want to employ me. But I came off them gradually and it was fine.

The course gave me the skills and tools, but more importantly the confidence to get back in the driver's seat of my own life. Exercise is now such a part of my life – I couldn't visualise my life without it now. Exercise is my medication now. Before I had back pain exercise wasn't something I ever really did. It didn't happen overnight – I had to keep challenging my thoughts and gradually I started to build my strength up and eventually after a while I was thinking of starting to work again. I started to slowly take some short trips – I still wasn't able to use public transport easily. I hadn't been on a train for donkey's years! Then after I'd been running my own programs to teach people about self management, I started to get invited to speak. I had to go to Madrid to speak at a conference in 1999 – that made me really challenge a whole lot of my fears about what I could and couldn't do. I look back on where I have come from – I used to be this frightened little guy and now last weekend I flew to Orlando in Florida for a weekend. I still have to keep challenging my thoughts.

After I finished the INPUT program, I went back and developed a 6 week course teaching the things that I had learned to people in the group who were interested. By then we had 700 members – but do you know how many people actually wanted to come on and do something to help themselves? Only 10! I knew I had to move on – they were frustrating me. So I left them to it – I think they met a few more times then it dissolved. I started up another support group, but you could only come to it if you had been on a rehab program or if you were going to do the 6 week course with me – I didn't want the "can't do" people mixing with the "can do" people.

I ran this 6 week course for next to nothing. I was teaching people the things that I had learnt about how to get better – needing to stay positive, about pacing, relaxation and all of that. Then I paid a physiotherapist to come in and teach the exercise components.

In 2000 I got a job for the Department of Health as a trainer. Our job was to help the local NHS clinics start to implement self management programs for chronic conditions. It was great – I was really motivated to get these programs up and running and even if I found people were blocking me, I was able to keep going. I got an award from the NHS for being persistent! I guess the work had meaning to me because I knew it was good – that it worked and it would help people.

Last year I was diagnosed with prostate cancer. I think having had the experience with the back pain in the past was helpful for me – it stopped me going too far down the path of the medical model in terms of being so attached to it all. It helped me to move into accepting it a bit quicker than I might have. I know that I have it and my levels are good now, but I also now that I just need to get on with it and live my life with it.

I think one of the good things that I have also learnt is that in dealing with my pain these days, I need to put my business head on – when you are making business decisions you need to be really objective and just make decisions without emotion. It's the same with pain – you need to be really objective about it and not use emotion so much – especially with flare ups. You need to just fall back on your plan, know that it will pass and not put your emotional head on. Pain doesn't scare me now like it used to.

Pete has a fabulous website which has wonderful resources for pain management www.paintoolkit.org

JOLETTA BELTON

My pain started just over seven years ago when I was working as a firefighter paramedic. It started with a routine medical call. It was about 1 o'clock in the morning and it was a cardiac arrest so it was a complicated case. We were in the emergency department and there was a lot of paperwork to fill out. Coming back out to the truck I realised I had left my clipboard in the hospital. I jumped down from the truck to go back in the hospital and I was in a hurry because I wanted everyone to get back to the station so that we could get some sleep. I missed the step on the cab and I went straight from the cab to the ground and twisted my hip. It wasn't that big of a deal. I was still able to run in and get the clipboard and get back to the truck. I could feel something at the time so I let my captain know. We filled out some paperwork because that was the regulations but I really wasn't worried about it at the time. It was 10 days later that I got to see the occupational doctor and he diagnosed it as a soft tissue injury. He assigned me to physical therapy and I went for a couple of weeks but the pain was getting worse. I was having trouble flexing my hip and getting up and down from the fire engine. By this stage the pain had been there for two months. Then I was called up for jury duty. Because I was a government employee we often had to do longer cases and in this case I was assigned to wrongful death trial. It required me to sit for really long time each day and I found it really uncomfortable and my pain escalated. It went on for a month. I went back to work after that and my pain levels were really high. I remember doing a training session one day that involved pulling hoses around as well as running up lots of stairs. I was finding the stairs really painful and I said to the captain that I was not really able to do it. That was the day that I realised I was becoming a hazard to my crew, to the public and to myself and I worried that if we got a big call, I wasn't going to be able to perform my duties. This was really difficult for me to admit because prior to the injury I was running and I had to do a lot of weight-lifting for my job. My partner at work at the time was 270 pounds with his kit on and I needed to be strong enough to be able to lift him if we were in a dangerous situation. I was running half marathons, going to the gym four days a week and lifting heavy weights. I was the fittest I had been in my life and I was in my early 30s. I had been with the fire department for seven years.

When I stopped work things started to fall apart

more. The pain was getting worse and without work and being in at the station I really lost my way. It hit me much harder than I though it would. Being a firefighter you tend to spend more time with your crew than you do with your family. The station really is a second home and you spend a good chunk of you life there. All of a sudden I wasn't doing that any more and it was a real sense of loss for me. Being a firefighter and being a problem solver I had a really hard time reaching out and asking for help. So I never called anybody and I never kept in contact with anybody. I lost contact with a lot of people in that time.

I had started physical therapy again and the pain just kept getting worse. Eventually I was sent to an orthopaedic surgeon and I had Cortisone injections into my hip. The pain got worse again after that and I saw another orthopaedic specialist who was a hip specialist. He diagnosed me with femoroacetabular impingement and I was so relieved because up until that point I had no answers for what was going on. When he proposed surgery I was really pleased because here was the answer to my problems – I thought it was all going to be over. I had a very biomechanics understanding of pain at that time and I thought that there was something very wrong with my tissues. He was a really wonderful guy – I felt like he was the first person who had really listened and understood me. I didn't do any of my own research about the surgery.

I felt like he cared so much and he took the time to talk to me and I felt tremendous relief and this was an answer – which set me up for greater disappointment because when he proposed it to the workers compensation agency they denied the claim and wouldn't pay for the surgery.

Being denied the surgery meant that I had to go through three medical review panels. It was an awful process – being on workers comp in general is awful. It would take so long to get a referral and then you would have to wait three months for the appointment because the doctors were so busy. I had been through this process a few times already so at the start of this panel process I knew that even if it did get approved, it was going to be a long time to subsequently get the appointment for the surgery. It is such a frustrating process. It was stressful and I felt like I was constantly fighting the system. Their goal seems to be to root out the fraudulent claims and this meant that you are always having to prove that you are in pain. I felt like I wasn't believed all the time.

I was eventually approved for surgery and I had that done 13 months after the initial incident of hip pain. After the surgery certain aspects of the pain went away – the really deep visceral components were completely gone, but I still had groin pain and sacroiliac joint pain. Up until this point I hadn't taken any pain relief and following the surgery I was also really adamant that I wouldn't take any narcotics or strong pain relief. I have a family history of addiction and I was really worried that if I took any of that, I would end up going down a wrong pathway. Knowing what I know now about pain science, I should have taken medication to get my pain better controlled following surgery. I realise how important that can be in preventing further persistent pain and in hindsight I could have taken that for a couple of weeks to better control that surgical pain. I just took the anti-inflammatories.

I was really wanting to get back to being active so I hit the physical therapy hard. I was weight bearing really early – It was all probably too much too soon and again, in hindsight I would have been a bit gentler with myself and allowed my body to heal and take it slow.

I still had pain though which was really frustrating because I was so sure that surgery was going to fix it for me. By six weeks my function was really improving and by 12 weeks I was going to the gym, doing big step ups at physical therapy and pushing it quite hard. The pain was there 24 hours a day and I was constantly worried because I was convinced that I had stuffed up my surgery – the pain was so bad that I just assumed that I had somehow ruined it and re-injured my hip.

I started trying other therapies like chiropractic, posture therapy and acupuncture. I would feel better temporarily but then the pain would come back. My physical therapist was finding it really difficult because she was working hard to really challenge me – my range of motion was fantastic and my strength was great – we speak about it now and she says that I was a big lesson to her about the idea that there is more to pain than just the biomechanics components.

Because I had already had surgery but still had pain, I was a problem for the workers compensation system – they don't handle this situation well. I really needed to be on light duties and I had to fight for that, but sitting was my worst position and gave me the most pain, so a normal desk job was out of the question. I couldn't even be in a car for five minutes at that time. My husband had to do all of our grocery shopping and other things like that for us. The drive up to work would have been 40 minutes and there was no way that I could do that, so I asked if I could work from home. They had been okay about me doing a desk job but they wouldn't let me work from home. During that time I had a battalion chief call me – he was someone that I considered a friend, I had been to his house and got on well with him – he essentially told me I was malingering and said that I was lying about not being able to drive. It was the most devastating thing that happened during the whole time – to be accused of lying by someone I really respected.

Eventually another chief who I really liked, fought for me and managed to get me a light duty assignment which was essentially at a different station. I could work from home and could report in once a week to the station. I was able to take the train up which meant that I could walk around during the trip and he was kind enough to pick me up from the train station.

I started working for the wellness and fitness coordinators office. I was having a really bad flare up of my pain – I hadn't slept for two weeks and I thought if I could just get a few more sessions of physical therapy then I could get this flare up under control. I rang the workers comp office and explained and they said that if I was in that much pain that I should just go to the emergency department and they denied the physical therapy. I was a former paramedic and I knew that that wasn't what the ED was for! It wasn't like I was trying to buck the system – I was trying to do whatever I could to stay at work! That was the start of my decision to leave the department altogether. I had been a good firefighter. I was good at my job and I had always done whatever they had asked me – being on committees, doing media appearances, training the rookie fire fighters. It was so disappointing and I felt like I was proving the people who believed that women didn't belong in the fire service. I felt like I was letting down all the other women who had to fight to be seen as a legitimate part of the fire department.

Three years to the day after I stepped off the rig and felt that twinge I medically retired from the fire department. Even that was a frustrating process because they won't let you out! I had to jump through all the hoops to actually be medically retired. It involved a process going through a quality medical board and they declared me medically unfit for work and signed all the paperwork.

I went back to school and began a degree in human movement and biomechanics. It involved a lot of sports and exercise psychology and that was where I started to learn more about a modern understanding of pain. I read the book "Explain Pain" by Lorimer Moseley and David Butler. Pain science was my research focus and it carried through all of our classes. School also gave me a label I could apply to myself because I was feeling really lost and didn't know who I was – at least with this I could call myself a student.

I wrote a lot of papers on pain science for assignments and gradually my understanding of pain started to turn around from one that was completely tissue and biome-chanically focused to one that understood that pain was far more complex and that how we understand our pain, our worries and thoughts have a big influence on pain. I was very fortunate to have the opportunity to interview Professor Moseley for a project. I spoke with him on Skype for 45 minutes and I had every pain science question I could put into that time. He was very gracious and patient and charismatic. At the end I asked him if he had one thing that he could sum up or recommend to people who are in pain and he answered "to love and be loved".

I was totally blown away – I was expecting a pain biology answer and that one sentence really flipped a switch in me – I was going about this wrong. I was so focused on what was wrong, what I had done to damage my tissues. It had sapped up all my energy and my resources. I had become so withdrawn from my family, friends and even my husband. Everything was pain – and it blinded me to everything else in my life. Probably with the context of the science I had been studying as well, the message started to sink in that my tissues were OK and that my pain was influenced by much more than just what was happening there. I wasn't doing any of my hobbies or movement any more. I hadn't wanted to move because I had those firmly held biomechanics beliefs that because it hurt when it moved it must be damaging the tissues and therefore it was bad. As my beliefs around those concepts loosened I realised that I could gradually start to get out there and do more. I was able to start thinking about my life again and not just thinking about my pain.

I also registered to go to the San Diego Pain Summit because Lorimer Moseley was going to be the keynote speaker. I felt like at that stage I had really understood the pain science but I couldn't really apply it to myself. It made sense on a different level and I think that was because I didn't really have anyone guiding me. Once I went to the Summit I felt like I had permission to really embrace this approach and get back to living my life. I knew that I didn't have all the answers but I was actually okay with that – I was learning that uncertainty is okay. I could focus on life and the things that were meaningful to me and not on the pain so much.

I started to go outside more – it was so simple! I had hardly been leaving the house until then, so I started just doing some neighborhood walks. At this time we moved to Colorado and was able to get out in nature more often – something that I had always loved but had completely stopped doing. I was walking and hiking gently and gradually started increasing the amount that I did. Being in nature also puts things in perspective. In the grand scheme of things this isn't that important. I also started the blog and started sharing my experiences with other people. Most importantly I started talking more about it with my husband. For so long I hadn't shared much of what was going on with my pain with him because we didn't know how to talk about it. I didn't want to burden or bore him with my problems and he didn't know how best to approach it. It was difficult! Talking about it with other people was fantastic for me as well because I didn't think that anybody else could understand what I had been going through. To find out that not only were lots of people having similar experiences but that they had the same thoughts and frustrations was a real revelation.

I made a decision to start reaching out to the friends and family who I had been disconnected to since the pain had started. I hadn't been able to talk to them about it and so I had to get better at having those conversations. I had to be able to say to people that this is what is going on and has been stopping me from being a part of your life, but I don't need you to fix it for me. I found out a lot of the time that people had stopped communicating with me because they felt helpless – they didn't know what to do to fix it.

My relationship with my husband had definitely suffered. We were able to just start talking about it more and discuss how both of us had been feeling. This stuff is hard because there is no manual for it! I didn't want to burden him and he didn't know how to fix me. I needed him to know that if I shared with him that I had a bad day with my pain, I just wanted him to kiss me on the head and say I'm sorry you had a bad day, and then fix dinner or do the washing – something practical to help me, rather than wanting to fix my pain. Once we started having these conversations everything changed.

For the friends and family the discussion went along the lines of me saying " this is what has been happening to me and I'm still here and I'm still the same person but things are just a little different regarding what I can do". Many of my friends were able to reconnect and re-establish a relationship with me. A few weren't and that was hard. Some of the conversations were really awkward – I hadn't returned their calls for many years.

At that time I was still in a lot of pain, especially with sitting. I was still very limited with what I could do. I had started to reconnect with people and I wanted to really get back to doing fun things. We had decided to go to a concert one night with a group of friends and my pain happened to be through the roof that night. I remember we were all standing there waiting for the band to start and I was just crying silent tears. My husband noticed and I said that I just really needed to go and lie down in the car. In the end everyone decided to leave the concert and I felt really bad – like I had ruined their night. After that, instead of giving up with trying to do new things like that, we just got smarter about how we planned it. We would make sure that I had my own car so I could leave if I needed to without disrupting other people and would try to reduce the time that I was out so it wasn't too long or too much sitting. It was a learning curve.

I eventually started flying to places and it was a terrifying prospect. I was so worried that I was going to flare it up and ruin the trip. I flew across the country for the first time and although I was miserable with the sitting, I also realised that I survived it, and the precious time that I got to spend with my family made it really worth it. In truth, the pain once I got there was no worse than how it was at home, so I reasoned that I might as well go and have fun and be around my family even if I was in pain. It became more about figuring out what I could do with pain, rather than trying to remove pain. I found that the more I engaged with my life, and doing things that were meaningful like going for hikes and hanging out with my friends, the more I became able to do those things with greater ease and the more my pain reduced. It was surprising! I had figured I was stuck with that level of pain for the rest of my life. I was finding that the more I did, the less pain I had, which was the opposite to what I had believed about my pain.

One of the other ways that I was able to stop focusing on my pain so much was taking photographs of nature. It was a new hobby that I could do and I could work within my own limitations. It also really helped me to appreciate the world – like I was seeing it through a new lens. It made me actually see the things around you rather than them just being a background. The other thing that really helped was volunteering. I was coaching people to learn to snowboard. I began doing it in small sessions on my own time. I was working with disabled athletes and paralympians who were training for Korea for the Olympics and with people with disabilities who were learning to snowboard. I think the volunteers got so much more out of it than the participants did. It helped shift my perspective and give me a broader understanding of how I wasn't the only one who suffered at times – people had cancer, disabilities, amputations and they also had pain and limitations and they got on with it anyway.

I don't know that any of this would have opened up for me if I hadn't come across the knowledge about pain. I think I would have still been stuck looking for an answer and a cure. Now my pain is almost non existent most days. Its not even something I really think about much.

Joletta writes a fantastic blog about pain and recovery. It can be found here: www.mycuppajo.com

J

I started getting back pain in about 2011. I was playing tennis pretty full on and also football. I was 16 at the time. The pain was pretty consistent but I was still able to run and play sports. It was more of a nuisance than anything else. That went on for a couple of years and I didn't do much about it. I went to see a couple of different physiotherapists and didn't have really good results. Because I was still able to do everything, my motivation to properly do something about it wasn't very high.

At the end of 2013, I had a fairly bad groin injury which I had just played with for the tail end of the footy season. After the season finished I decided that I needed to rest the injury to let it heal and it was when I took that time off that my back started to get really bad. When I tried to return the back pain would flare up and it got to a point where I really couldn't run for more than 100 metres.

Around this time I had a few scans and went to see a musculoskeletal physician. The scans showed I had a bit of a scoliosis and also a partial sacralisation of my lowest lumbar vertebrae which they thought could be the source of the pain. They weren't 100% sure that it was the cause – they told me that they don't always cause pain, but it was the first thing that had actually showed up.

At this time the pain was really interfering with my life. I was working as a waiter in a cafe and being on my feet all the time was a real struggle. Sitting at uni was also tough – doing exams and sitting in lectures was really uncomfortable. I tried some anti-inflammatories which didn't help much. I also had some cortisone and local anaesthetic injections into the facet joints and into the regions where I was getting the pain. It didn't help at all and after the third one failed I was pretty much ready to give up. The way the doctor had spoken about it had really got my hopes up and so I was really upset when it didn't work. It was such an emotional rollercoaster. After that the doctor was out of ideas and he suggested trying a new physiotherapist. By that stage I had seen a chiropractor and even a podiatrist to see if it was coming from my feet. The pain was getting worse.

I felt fairly defeated and I didn't want to try any more treatments. I was prepared to just learn to live with it day to day and I was ready to give up on sport. I hadn't played for 2-3 years by this stage. I knew my chances of reaching my goals to play really high level tennis – (I had wanted to see if I could get on the tour or at the least play college tennis) were over because I was too old. I missed the fun bits of playing footy too – the social side of things.

My mum convinced me to keep trying to find someone who could help me. I felt really guilty because she was spending all this money on medical appointments and it wasn't helping. I also didn't really want to get my hopes up again and go through that sense of defeat with another round of failed treatments. I thought that I could just learn to live without sport. Mum knew how much I enjoyed playing sport and also said that I needed to do something about it because it was going to interfere with other areas of my life.

Mum brought me to see an osteopath and she explained a lot about the pain – she drew diagrams and it made a lot of sense to me. Overall I think the message was that the pain didn't mean that there was anything actually wrong with my spine. She started me with another osteopath at the same time who was getting me started in the gym. I really liked this part because it was structured and was getting back to doing what I enjoyed. I don't think I really even noticed that I was getting better – I was just so focused on achieving what he had set for me and gradually I started getting stronger and was just more able to do things. Pretty soon he had me running on the treadmill in short bursts and then before I realised, I was running for 10 minutes at a time. I hadn't been able to run at all for nearly three years prior to that.

Even though I was making big progress at the gym and with the running, I didn't feel like I was getting better because I still had pain. I didn't really see it as success because I don't think I knew what point I wanted to get back to. I was annoyed about losing athleticism, speed and explosiveness. I had to learn to adjust to this being my new normal.

There were times when my osteopaths would be so excited about the improvement and I just wouldn't feel that happy about it. There was one time when I was talking with the first osteopath about how I had played tennis with my Dad for 40 minutes on the weekend. This was pretty much only a month into the treatment. I had built up from hitting a ball against the wall and then was able to have a hit with Dad. She thought it was fantastic but all I could think of was "What is the point?" Because I had always played at such as high level, it had been really hard to watch other people at my level keep progressing and I couldn't do anything about it. So my success of just having a hit didn't really seem like a win to me – even though it was something I wouldn't have been able to do a month before that. I felt like I had gone backwards so much that having a casual hit wasn't worth celebrating.

They sent me to a sports doctor for another opinion and also just to have a doctor on the team who was treating me. He put me on some endep (a medication frequently used in persistent pain) which didn't really help.

He also referred me to a sports psychologist. I found it pretty unnatural talking about my feelings. I told her about how I wanted to quit and how I didn't see much point unless I could get back to where I had hoped to be. I expected her to give more wise advise – she didn't really say much but the best thing about it was, the bits that she did say, really made me think. Most of the benefit I got from that was actually after the sessions, when I would be going over it in my mind. I think I got a lot of clarity around some of those issues and it was helpful.

I was really committed at this point, especially after I started running because I could see that it was possible to actually get back to footy. The timeline was pretty helpful because I knew that if I kept improving I could do a pre-season later that year and start back at football. I was training 4 times a week. I kept building up and then I started back at footy. I told the coaches that I had some issues with my back so that he understood if I had to stop. I didn't do full training sessions to start but then I worked up to it. I had to re-invent myself a bit and play a different position because I had lost a lot of that explosive speed but I had also put on more muscle.

My back pain now doesn't really bother me. If I haven't slept or I'm stressed it does give me a niggle but on the whole it isn't a big deal. It occasionally bothers me but not enough to do anything about. I don't see myself as someone with a back problem now but for a long time

I was "the guy with the back problems". Mum is pretty happy with how it all turned out. She takes this stuff to heart and she wanted the best for me.

R

I had always loved exercise and had a habit of always pushing myself very hard. I loved things like aerobics classes where they really encouraged you to thrash yourself! I would really get into it. The first time that I felt something wrong with my leg was when I was training harder than I was ready for and essentially gave myself an overuse type of injury in my hamstring. I was 21 at the time and studying finance at university. Pretty much from that time on I have had some sort of issue with that hip region of my body. I had a lot of on and off types of injuries which didn't always stop me from doing things – I would always be pushing right to the edge of that injury and never let it properly recover. By the time I was 23 I was doing some long distance running – up to 18 km runs, and I was also doing a lot of study as I was doing my masters. I noticed at around this time that I had a pinching pain in my hip when I was sitting. I didn't know what it was and I saw a couple of physiotherapists. It was a hard pain to pin down. I had a few scans and no one really could tell me what was wrong or how to fix it. I was really frustrated because I didn't like not being in control of it.

A physiotherapist at the time mentioned femoro-acetabular impingement syndrome and I latched onto that as a possible answer – I spent a lot of time researching it online and the symptoms that they described seemed to fit what I was going through. I went on a four year journey from that point of pursuing a surgical solution to this problem that I was convinced that I had. My understanding of the condition was that there was something wrong with my hip – that something was impinging in my hip and that was causing the pain. I believed that if I could just get someone to remove the impingement, the pain would go away.

I spent a lot of time online and looking for word of mouth recommendations to find the best orthopaedic surgeon to do the surgery for me. The first surgeon that I went to agreed with my diagnosis and went ahead with the surgery. I remember quite clearly the test that they did to determine the presence or absence of impingement, which was to rotate your hip in a particular way, seemed to me to be very subjective. I also got the impression from him that he was never certain or convinced that this was definitely what was going on. The day after the surgery he repeated the test and I felt like the way that he responded to the outcomes of the test following surgery was not positive. He was not emphatic that it had actually "worked" and I was probably reading a lot into his reaction to the testing following surgery. He was also very vague about what he had actually done, what had been going on and if the surgery had been a success. There was never really clear pathology around the impingement – the CT and MRI had shown virtually nothing but these subjective tests had shown that it was present. I was aware of this at the time but I was reassured that the surgeons were confident that there was a problem they could fix. I was also impatient and a quick fix was exactly what I was after. So when afterwards, he wasn't showing confidence that the surgery had changed these subjective tests, I felt less confident this was going to fix the problem. I was really upset. I didn't get much better with that pain following the surgery.

I was able to get back to running but not to the volume that I had been able to before the surgery. At this time I moved to Melbourne and changed jobs. I saw a new physiotherapist there and he gave me a lot of exercises to do at home. They were really difficult to do because there was too many of them and I didn't trust that they were going to help so I ended up stopping doing them. I was stressed at my new job and spending a lot of time sitting. I was also a bit lonely because I didn't know anyone and my boyfriend was overseas.

I was getting really fed up with not being better and

wanting to get back to where I was prior to it all starting. I could only really run 5 kms and that wasn't good enough for me. I did some online research and tried to find a new person to help. I looked for the best person for this condition in Melbourne and found a well respected physiotherapist and went along to see him. He was very certain, without seeing any scans but based on these same subjective tests, that I needed further surgery because the first one hadn't worked. He was aggressively confident about this and his confidence and certainty convinced me that this was the best step forward, so I made an appointment with the surgeon he was suggesting. Because I was away from home and no one was around to support me, I was making these decisions on my own. In a way, I wish I had someone who was able to go over it with me and perhaps apply the brakes a bit! I was so hell bent on finding that quick fix that I was going to believe anyone who fed into that narrative and dismiss information on other approaches like rehab. In hindsight I was pretty vulnerable.

When I went for that second surgery it was two years after the first surgery. Because of the research I had done and also because of the high praise from the physiotherapist, I believed this surgeon was the best in the game. Following the surgery I took the recommended three weeks off after surgery and went back to that same physiotherapist for rehab.

When I went back to work I was assigned to a really important project finance transaction. The director who I was working under was very condescending and put a lot of pressure on me. I became really obsessed with detail in the work which meant that I was slow to produce the work. I felt like I was disappointing him which made me more anxious, which made me more focussed on the detail and highly stressed. It became a vicious cycle.

Because we were doing massive days I was spending up to 14 hours a day sitting, wasn't able to fit in the rehab and even was catching taxis home because the company paid for it on those late nights. Putting this all together, along with the stressful environment, my hip pain got worse and worse. It started to go down my leg and it was later diagnosed as being neuropathic pain. I went back to the physiotherapist and described to him what was happening and his response was that I needed surgery again. I lost it at that point. I felt like he had no idea what he was talking about and I was angry. I had trusted that he had the answers and he had let me down. I was overwhelmed with despair after walking away from that appointment. I had spent so much money, so much time, taken time off work and things were just getting worse.

I knew that sitting made the pain worse. I also knew that in order to finish this particular task, but also in general my job, I needed to spend a lot of time at my desk sitting. I felt trapped because I knew it was making me worse but also the pain was distracting me, making work harder and me less efficient. I was becoming very aware of what people were saying about my work and my efforts.

I asked for a standing desk because I thought that might be helpful. We had to get a corporate injury management team involved in order to approve the workplace changes. It was such an awful experience to have to go through – it seemed like their job was to minimise costs and therefore they intention was to block any changes. We had meetings where they would just question me and my directors all about my pain and why it was absolutely necessary for me to have a standing desk. Some of my superiors were really wanting to help and suggested that I just take the corporate credit card and purchase a standing desk from Officeworks. Unfortunately though because the process was underway we had to go through the proper channels. In one of these meetings I was almost hysterical trying to describe how the more I sat the worse my pain was and that it was meaning that I just couldn't do my job. There was just no empathy or understanding from their point of view.

The end result of all of these meeting was that instead of getting a standing desk which was the simplest solution, I was told that I needed to take leave from work. I took all of my annual leave because there was a view that potentially it would get better if I took a break. I also took unpaid leave and was off for a total of 6 weeks.

I remember being at home and being bored. I became totally focussed on the pain because I had nothing else to think about – is it better today? Is it worse today? I continued my search to find the perfect physiotherapist or doctor who was going to have the answers. One of the doctors that I went to see had chastised me about the fact that I had gone for a 5 km walk and had pain afterwards – he said that it was silly of me to go for such a long walk and expect to be ok. It just added to the confusion as to whether I should be resting or not.

I found another physiotherapist who suggested that the problem was in my nervous system and labeled it as chronic pain. I really didn't want to hear that message because it didn't fit with my idea that something was still wrong in my hip.

At this time my research for my pain had directed me towards a pain specialist. I was again hoping that there was going to be a procedure that could be done to switch off the pain. He told me that I couldn't have an invasive procedure as it was unlikely to work. He prescribed Lyrica and told me that it was unlikely that the pain would go away. He said that with a combination of mindfulness, addressing depression, getting stronger, seeing a psychologist, having the standing desk and with time, it would be likely that the pain would drop down but would actually never go away. In hindsight that message was so spot on and is pretty much how things have turned out

– but again, at that time, it just wasn't the message that I was wanting to hear.

On his recommendation I started seeing a pain psychologist who was fantastic. At the same time I was also seeing a myotherapist who understood a lot about chronic pain and while she was working on my hip and back we spent a lot of time talking. I developed a really good rapport with her and she gently started to tell me similar messages to what that last physiotherapist had said. After four sessions she loaned me the book Explain Pain and I read it at home. It felt right for me – everything in it described my situation. I felt really sad reading it because it made me reflect on the last four years of what I had been going through. At the same time though it gave me hope because I could see that there was a way forward. It was just that it was a different and contrasting message to the one I had been so focussed on for the last four years.

At this time I was transitioning back to work and that same team who had assessed me for the standing desk had mandated that I return to work really gradually and on a plan so I was doing half days and only working a few days a week to begin with. They also still were being difficult with the standing desk – after all that. I ended up actually just going and buying it myself with the corporate credit card after my boss told me again to just do it.

My confidence was really rocked when I started back at work. I was convinced on one level that I just wasn't going to be able to do this work in the long term. I needed to break up the day by going for short walks so that I wasn't sitting too long. Some of my bosses were really unsupportive and suggested that I consider other careers. I had convinced myself that the long hours and the stress of that job was going to mean that I couldn't continue.

We had a restructure and I had a new director who was completely encouraging and said things along the lines of – you are valuable to us whether you are working three days a week or five, we can find things for you to do and you don't need to think about leaving. He said that I was an asset even if I wasn't working full time It was like a watershed moment for me. To have that back up from a senior figure was so comforting because up until that point I was seeing myself as a burden. I knew that they couldn't fire me and I was so worried about that other people were judging me – seeing me as a someone who was a "bludger". (Australian slang for someone who is lazy and tries to get out of work)

After that boost in my confidence I felt so much better within myself and fairly quickly was able to get back to full time work. I had spent most of that year either off work or working part time. Once I had the standing desk it made working so much easier – something so simple but it made the difference between being able to work or not work.

My work with the psychologist was really helping me

to get over all my worries about being judged and about some unhelpful thoughts that I had regarding how I viewed myself as successful or a failure at work. I think at that time she saved my life. Just before that director had boosted my confidence by saying that I was an asset and they wanted me to stay, I had been having occasional suicidal thoughts . She helped me to address the depression and helped to link me in with a good doctor to help manage the medication side of things. She was really caring and got me through those dark times.

The Lyrica really helped me to be able to cope with the pain at work and I was coasting along and gradually building up. At that time I had been recommended a new osteopath who was running a persistent pain program. It was largely talking about the condition and it focused on moving forward and adapting to the pain, rather than focusing on getting rid of it. We looked at all the things that I hadn't been able to do because of the pain and we worked out ways that I could get back to doing them, even if it was only in tiny amounts. Things like going to the movies, riding my bike and getting back to yoga. It was a different focus to everything that I had done before and obviously I was in the right headspace to hear that message – the pain doesn't have to have as much meaning and it doesn't have to completely go away for me to live my life. We did lots of planning so that I could achieve some of these things – for example I found the TENS machine to be really helpful for short term discomfort, so when I planned to go the movies for the first time, I made sure I had the TENS all set up, was able to get up and go for a short walk without making too much fuss. I also had a "get out" plan so that I knew I could leave if things were getting too much. That first time I tried it out, I ended up watching two movies in a row! There was probably so much fear around actually doing it, that when I had all these safety plans in place, I obviously felt a lot more relaxed and was able to do it. I tried to make sure that I was doing fun stuff more often and the way we approached it was structured and pragmatic. It just worked for me. These things started to make me feel more normal because I think deep down, that was what had been bugging me – "normal" people didn't have to think about getting on a short plane trip and "normal" people didn't have to think about work functions that involved too much sitting. Doing some of these things made me feel normal again, and that took a lot of the fear and power of the pain away. My fear of having pain and my need for it to completely go was probably really centered around the worry that it was going to impact on my life. When I started to prove to myself that it didn't have to, it just started to become less of a frightening thing.

We also spent a lot of time talking about the idea that being in the pain zone was not the end of the earth. I realised that I could react differently to the presence of pain, and that for example, if it started to bother me in the movie, instead of freaking out, I could just recognise that it was there, it is what it is, and I am enjoying the movie and being out with my friend. It made me realise that I didn't have to be black and white about the pain – that sometimes, in pursuing the stuff that gave me joy and made me feel normal, a little bit of pain was okay. I was making a choice to be in that situation and I accepted that a bit of pain might be inevitable but it was worth it. It was different to my previous mindset where I was constantly looking to avoid or remove the pain completely. I wanted to live a normal life and sometimes doing that meant that there might be bad days. Its largely based around acceptance and commitment therapy or ACT.

I also knew that in doing some of these activities that could potentially aggravate my pain, that I had some control over how I dealt with those flare ups – I had a small bag of tricks if you like! I knew that the TENS machine worked well for times like that, I was able to adjust my dose of Lyrica if the pain was worse for a short while, I could try mindfulness as that also helped and sometimes gentle stretching could help. Knowing all of this was there as a backup, and also knowing that the pain didn't mean that something was wrong, I was gradually able to just get back to doing pretty much everything. I got back to "normal"

To get physically stronger I worked with a trainer who

helped me to use a graded approach to progressively get stronger. It was such a hard process because I was so used to going hard and pushing myself and this was really strict with the progressions. It felt slow and useless in the beginning. I found this fairly quickly raised my pain thresholds and I was getting less pain overall. I started running again using this approach, just doing really small amounts at a time – I was running less than a minute a time on the treadmill. Within about 5 months I was invited by friends to run a 10Km run at the Melbourne Marathon Event and was able to do that without flaring up which really surprised me.

I continued to get stronger and gradually brought my Lyrica down. I had some difficulty getting off the antidepressants and ended up having to go back on them and try coming off them again later but much slower than I had the first time.

I was going really well overall – I was managing really well without the antidepressants and without the Lyrica. I was exercising and work was great. Overall, the hip was just not much of a problem for me, when in the years prior to that, it had been my central focus, the thing that defined me.

I have had one time when the pain has come back and bothered me – I moved to France to finish my Masters degree and found myself stressed, lonely, it was winter and I was not able to keep running for exercise because I had sprained my ankle. I was quite amazed at how quickly the pain started to bother me and also how depressed I got. I was able to recognise it pretty quickly, I got back onto some medication and when I eventually returned to Melbourne, I was able to get back in control of it again. I am not sure that it will ever completely leave me and sometimes I get sad about the journey and the sadness that it took me on. I'm so glad that I was able to hear that message that several of the practitioners were telling me – to be able to get off that search for the answers and realise that there were no easy answers and I didn't need to be so afraid of pain.

BEN

I was an elite junior footballer and after playing a good season at 16 years old I started to realise with advice from those around me that I could probably make a career out of being a professional Australian Rules Football player. I was in year 11 at the time and really dedicated myself to football. My studies suffered for it but I didn't worry too much because I knew I was going to be a footballer. I went from one season and kept training right into the preseason of the next so I didn't really have a break. My training load increased a lot, probably a bit too much and a bit too fast, which is a common thing for young footballers. It was a really hot year and the grounds were very hard. I started to develop some groin pain. It was on both sides and generally around the pubic bone. That began the search for answers – I needed to find out what was wrong.

I kept on training and pushing it, trying to ignore it and then it reached a point where I couldn't keep doing that. So I stopped completely and I was diagnosed with osteitis pubis which was a very popular diagnosis at the time. I began seeing some physiotherapists and I didn't always do what they suggested. I trusted them and had a good rapport. I felt like they were doing the right things for me.

I missed the whole of my top age season of football with groin pain which had started as acute and localised and then over the year it spread and became more diffuse. The physiotherapists sent me to a sports physician who sent me for a lot of scans. At them time there were some things showing up on the scans but my caregivers interpreted those findings differently – some thought they meant a lot, others didn't. There were some changes at the pubic symphysis and I really focused on that. I decided that was my problem and I was awfully good at convincing those around me to also focus on that. I convinced my parents to pursue that pathway and also was eager to go along with caregivers who were suggested an answer or a solution to the problem. I was frustrated and upset and just wanted to get better so I would hone in on that intervention and push for it to be done.

The first intervention suggested after a couple of cortisone injections was to have an adductor release on both sides – the intention is to cut the tendons and reduce the tension on the pubic region. I wanted to see the absolute best surgeon so I flew up to Sydney which was a big deal. I had been in pain for about 10 months by this time and unfortunately it didn't produce any results. I still had pain. I still wasn't playing footy. I had been told I would be back playing in 8 weeks and the pain got worse instead of better. I got to a point where it was so sore that I couldn't wear clothes that were tight around that region – couldn't wear tight underwear or anything else that was touching that area. It was so sensitive. I was trying hard to do the rehab but I still couldn't run and couldn't kick a ball so I was getting really frustrated.

There was also pressure from the clubs because I was taking up a spot for the junior elite players and they were supporting me. In the back of my mind I knew that time was ticking – I had to get better if I wanted to keep my spot and be able to play at that top level. I was also doing my final year of high school and was finding it difficult to study both because of the pain and because I didn't care too much about school because I was still convinced that I was going to be a footballer.

I realised that that it wasn't getting any better and I saw a different surgeon in Melbourne for another opinion. They suggested that I have a pubic symphysis clearance operation. I went ahead with that and it was about 10 months after the first surgery. It was the most painful operation of any that I had. The area was already super sensitive. The surgeon said because I was going to have a bit of time off anyway (he was suggesting that I would need 3 months before I could play) that I also have hip arthroscopy to remove a cam and also fix a tear in my hip capsule. I had this done 2 weeks after the pubic symphysis clearance. I had asked what he thought the success rates of the surgery would be and he said confidently that it would be 95-98% success rate. This was similar to the odds the first surgeon had given me and at that time I wasn't jaded enough to be skeptical!

During the surgery they didn't find the cam impingement was causing a problem like they thought it might have been according to the MRI. They removed the cam and fixed the small labral tear. The pain after that first pubic symphysis surgery was awful. I couldn't laugh, sneeze or even talk loudly for a long time – nearly a year after the surgery because of the attachment of the abdominal muscles onto that area. It was so much pain. I was taking a lot of anti-inflammatory medication but never any opioids.

I took a gap year after year 12 to focus my energies on my body and my football. Early on in this part of my rehab I was really excited. I had all these promises that it was going to go well. I was also put in touch with an AFL player who had just had the same surgery done and was going really well. He was very encouraging so I was pretty excited. I felt like I had a new groin. I was working with both the club physiotherapist and another physiotherapist outside of the club – I believe at the time he was the most expensive physiotherapist in the country! There was a lot of focus on core stability, bracing every time you moved and there was a lot of deep tissue massage which aimed to break up scar tissue. Now, as a physiotherapy student myself I can see that these treatments were probably really unhelpful – the bracing was pulling on the already sensitised pubic regions and the deep tissue massage was just causing more pain to an already sore area – we know that breaking up scar tissue is just nonsense now – but I understand that both of those were thought to be the right things to do at that time. As time passed and I was failing to meet the milestones that were projected for me I started to get frustrated. I was wondering what was happening. I went back to see the sports physicians – I hopped around between practitioners because I was good at getting what I wanted out of them, and also selling that idea to my parents who were funding all of the treatments.

At this time I left the football club that I had been with because I hadn't yet played a game for them and they were no longer willing to keep me at the club. I started playing for a different club who were in the VFL. They were a great bunch of people. I made some great friends and did a lot of rehab with their team with the idea that I would get better and eventually be able to play for them. I was three years into the journey and was still very narrowly focussed on becoming a professional player. Even after being dropped by the other club, I still felt there was hope and it was still the driving force for me.

I was studying a bachelor of exercise science at university and was training and as there were more signs that this career in football might not eventuate, I started having some mental health problems. It started to effect my studies whereas it previously hadn't – I'd been a really happy kid through year 12.

I had a further surgery to try to release the adductors again. I then had prolotherapy, PRP injections, loads of cortisone injections, the works. At the start of having all of these interventions and surgeries I felt excited going into them thinking that this could help or that this might be the one. As I went along the journey I became more skeptical – I realised these interventions weren't helping.

By this stage I was moving like a crab. I had to shuffle to get around. I started skipping classes, I stopped hanging out with friends as much and my mental health deteriorated. Anything that I thought might impact negatively on my rehab I would avoid. This meant that I wouldn't play backyard cricket if the boys were playing, or if they were going out drinking I wouldn't go out because I didn't want to be standing around all night. I was really fearful about movement, even with things like mowing the lawns.

I started seeing a psychologist at that time. I had started to recognise that I was depressed. She thought that I was grieving for the loss of my dreams. I don't think I was ready to hear that message. I was in denial. I don't think the approaches she was using were very up to date or appropriate. It probably helped a bit. She suggested that I try some antidepressants which I started to take and then decided that I didn't want to continue them so I stopped after a week before they would have had a chance to do anything. I was having massive mood swings. I would get really angry and was really good at smashing things. I would have these melt downs about once every two weeks. We have a gym out the back of our house and I would go out there and smash things up. I would never let these feelings spill over in social circumstances – I would only let it out at home.

I had built my identity around being an elite athlete for the length of my late teens and early twenties so when that didn't eventuate I kind of lost a sense of identity. Over this four year journey I had only played one game of football. The club asked me to drop back to a local club and return if I was able to get to a level that was good enough for their level. They were basically saying that they had had enough of keeping me on their books. It was devastating. I was 21 at that stage and was still in a lot of pain. 6 years of my life had been consumed and I think about how much money and heartache my parents had spent on me. I couldn't go to watch a game of local footy because I just couldn't be around it and I couldn't stand everyone asking me how I was going. I got sick of getting advice from everyone. I got pretty bitter because by this stage many of the guys I had started with in the earlier days had gone on to be drafted into the League and were playing professional footy.

I had spent a lot of time on a bike in the gym and my sister was also an elite cyclist at the time. I decided to buy myself a good bike and started riding more. I enjoyed it and was getting good at it. I made some good friends to ride with and the focus came off the football a bit which was probably a good thing. I got good quite quickly on the bike and ended up sort of being faced with the same dilemma. People were encouraging me to strive to get into competitive cycling, and I knew I probably could do it physically but I also knew that I didn't want to put myself back through that again. The injuries and the potential failures. I didn't think I could cope.

Because a lot of the pressure around football had come off, I found I was able to run a bit and also to kick the footy around a bit. I had finished my degree and was less stressed overall. I had less pain in general. I got an offer to play for a country football club, a club that had been trying to get me to play for three years. They offered quite a good pay deal and so I decided to give it a go. I met my current physiotherapist at that time and he is amazing. I worked with him for 6 months in the lead up to that season. I really trusted him and at the same time I was starting to learn about pain. My sister had been concurrently going through her own pain journey – a back injury had interrupted her training for over a year and she had got back into it with the help of good clinicians and the book Explain Pain. She lent it to me because she thought it would really help me. The book made sense to me. I started learning more and more about pain science – I read every blog, listened to every podcast I could get my hands on. I think if Lorimer Moseley's YouTube videos have about a million views on each of them, about half a million of them are mine! Together with this new understanding of pain, the physiotherapist and the training, I started to do really well. The explanations in the book helped me to understand why my physiotherapist was taking my rehab so slowly. It was such a frustrating process but I understood why he was using those graded exposure principles and why he was only adding 50 meters to my running each week.

My physiotherapist sent me to the sports doctors within his clinic because he thought that we should take a co-ordinated, team approach to get me on the field and that some medication may help us to get there. They started treating me with some Pregabalin which I trained on for most of the pre season. It helped me to be able to do what I did but it is such a terrible drug. Honestly, I couldn't put together a sentence or wake up properly until about midday the whole time I was on it . I didn't like the drugs but I recognised they were helping me and that they didn't have to be forever. I stopped taking them once I started playing.

I had enrolled in a masters of teaching and also started playing for the country team. The football was terrible! I played some good football and then I played some really average football. In hindsight, I don't know how I thought I could have not played at all for four years and then just expected to be good at it! I felt the external pressure from the club to play well because they were paying me. Every few weeks I would pull out a good game and that would keep them happy. I met some great guys on the team and got to know them well on the weekly bus trips up there. I was still sore. After each game I couldn't move or run from the Sunday through till later in the week. Usually by Thursday I could start to train a little bit. I was really hurting but I would treat it like a job and I would put the time into it to get through. I would do a lot of rehab work and would see the physiotherapist twice a week between games. I was progressing. I think if I had continued along that path I would have come good within a year or so. It definitely wasn't the best way to go about it. I was skipping a lot of steps for a graded exposure approach and pushed through too much pain. Its amazing what a carrot on a stick being paid to play became. But about halfway through the year I realised that I didn't want to play football anymore! I'd finally got to the point where I could play football and I realised that I didn't want to play football. I had been enjoying the riding so much more. I played out the rest of the year and continued to improve with movement. I was less fearful of pain. I was getting much stronger.

I became a teacher and at the same time began enjoying exercise and movement. It was more about fun and being social rather than being a chore. I loved running around with the kids at school. I met some great colleagues at the school and my focus in life really expanded from being so narrow and all about football, to being more about living life. I felt like I had come out of a dark tunnel. Pain just wasn't on my radar so much. It didn't consume me like it had and that constant desire and search to be out of pain had gone away.

One of the key things that I take away from my story is that you really need to be putting your focus on other areas. It's hard. It is so hard. You need to not close yourself in.

I still have some restrictions in my range of motion in my hip. I know how to manage my training loads – I know if I spike my loads too much I will flare it up but I understand that and I don't get worried about it.

I enjoyed the teaching but my heart wasn't 100% in it. I decided to apply for physiotherapy and was lucky enough to get a spot in the course. The other students are sick of hearing about me banging on about pain science already. I believe they are teaching it well so far, but I don't think there is anywhere near enough emphasis on what pain is and how a biopsychosocial approach works.

It needs to be taught to students from day one. I hope that one day Explain Pain Supercharged will be the platform textbook for all health courses.

LOU

I've had migraines for as long as I can remember, however, they weren't diagnosed as migraines until my mid-twenties. I have clear memories as young girl, several times a year, lying in bed for a couple of days at a time, vomiting and feeling awful with a severe left-sided head pain and sensitivity to movement and light. By the time I went to university a migraine would happen after exams or some major assessment. I would end up in bed for two, three or maybe even 4 days. I would vomit and I just wanted to stay in bed until it was over. I had great friends who would drop in to check on me. As I just accepted this was part of my life I never worried too much about it but it did mean that while everybody else was off partying or living a normal life, I missed out.

I moved to Sydney to do a Ph.D. and my migraines became more frequent and started to really interfere with my life. This was especially so when a migraine begun just before Christmas and I realized that I wouldn't to be able to drive to Melbourne for the family Christmas.

I didn't know what to do so I went to see my doctor who told me it was a migraine and said he would give me some medication to get rid of it but it would really knock me out. My professor took me home and I woke up the next day with no migraine and that changed my life because I realised that I could actually stop this thing with this concoction of drugs - a combination of pethidine (opioid), dexamethasone (steroid), and maxolon (for nausea). The medication took 12 hours to cure the migraine because that's how long it took for the dexamethasone to kick in. Looking back, that was also where I was set on that path whereby I needed those drugs to survive my migraines.

Each time I had a migraine from then on, my doctor would treat me with the same concoction of drugs. We tried the usual migraine preventatives but nothing worked. He sent me to see a specialist who was said to be a guru of migraines who said that all I needed to do was continue with the concoction of drugs because they seemed to be working which left me feeling very despondent.

In the years that followed I saw many specialists but I felt like I was put in the too hard basket because the conventional migraine treatments failed to work with me. I become very aware of the fact that I was reliant on other people when I had a migraine because I needed someone to drive me to the doctor and then bring me home. These friends were shocked when they saw the state I was in and the effect of the drugs. I knew that this wasn't normal but I always thought that I could get over it and find a cure for it. At that stage I was finished my Ph.D. and had moved to a different university to take up a lectureship. Though I rarely had to cancel a lecture I regularly had to get a friend to take me to the doctor after a lecture.

On the most exciting day of your life - your wedding day, of course I got a migraine. I managed to get through most of the wedding but had to leave towards the end of the dinner. I don't think many people noticed but of course I remember. I missed out on so many things but I just learnt to accept that this is what happens to me and was grateful it wasn't something worse.

I moved to Canberra and got a new doctor. Shortly after that I got pregnant and I didn't have a migraine for the whole nine months. After my son was born, the migraines returned. I was determined to breastfeed and I worked with the lactation consultants determine the timing and frequency of feeds so that I could keep feeding without exposing him to harmful doses of the medication when I had a migraine.

My doctor and her colleagues were amazing – they really cared for me and kept trying different approaches. I was getting migraines about once a week at that stage and then I got pregnant with my second son. Unfortunately I had migraines all through that second pregnancy and there was a lot of concern around the baby being exposed to the drugs so they monitored him very closely. Unexpectedly I became pregnant a third time. Both my husband and my doctor thought that I should have a termination because of the impact of the migraines and drugs on me and the baby. It was such an incredibly difficult decision for all of us but I decided go ahead with the pregnancy.

I often think back to the type of mother I was back then. I could get the kids to school most days and I could pick them up maybe three days a week but the other days I needed friends to pick them up, or I would have to get my husband to take time off work. He would have to cook dinner or friends would cook dinner for us. I was relying on so many people. The saddest part for me was that frequently my infant son would have to be looked after by someone else. I would breastfeed him but then other people would look after him. My children don't remember any of this, but I do.

It was a really hard time. The doctors at the surgery were really aware of what was happening and were very supportive and helpful. They could see that if I didn't have my husband, Mike, the situation wouldn't be sustainable. He had a flexible job and there were many times when I would have to call him in the middle of the day and he would have to leave work to come and take me to the doctor and then to pick up the boys. The other consequence of this was that the kids were often being dragged to after-hours doctors. We had a letter from my treating doctor and we also carried the medication with us. Most doctors either knew of situation or were understanding when they read the letter, however, some doctors refused treatment because of the pethidine.

Traveling was a really big problem because I couldn't go anywhere without knowing that I could get someone to administer the drugs. We planned a trip Cape York which is very isolated and we knew it could be a problem if I got a migraine. We asked our doctor if she would teach Mike to administer the drugs. She was hesitant as this meant handing over the control of opioids to my husband. She felt this was ethically undesirable because it put him in an awkward position however she did consent. The trip went well despite several migraines which Mike was able to treat.

At this point my doctor decided to send me to a well-known researcher and professor in Sydney who specialised in problematic migraines. At the first visit I went through my history with him, 'Prof'. Prof concluded the consultation by saying he wasn't very hopeful which made me feel terrible as we had put all our hope in him. On my return to Canberra I told my doctor that I was never going back to Prof yet she was quite firm with me and said that he was our only hope and that we had to at least give it a try.

People who were close to me would look at my life

and wonder how I managed to keep going through it all. I had a group of families who were very close to me and cared for me. If we didn't have that support network of people who never questioned me I wouldn't have coped. My husband was fantastic and my doctor never gave up hope. I was really well supported. People on the outside wouldn't really see how bad it was. They would see me without a migraine and they wouldn't really know what was going on. I was always really positive but occasionally it would really get me down.

Prof put me on a combination of Endep and Topamax. These drugs didn't really change the frequency of the migraines but he wanted me to be stabilized on those these before he begun any other treatment. By this time the pethidine was not very helpful and the dexamethasone was causing some problems. I had started to put on a lot of weight with swelling and fluid and also my bone density had started to reduce. I found both of these made me sleepy and it affectedly memory and cognition. After two years under Prof's care he admitted me to hospital as an inpatient where I was given a local anaesthetic infusion for 2 weeks as well as Botox injections. I had several teams looking after me - one was the drug addiction team to deal with the opioids. It was hard being treated like a drug addict. Another team was to deal with the steroids and another team was the pain management team. The infusion worked well and I immediately felt better however once I returned home I fell back into the same migraine pattern as before.

Prof decided to repeat the infusion and I got a sense that he wasn't going to give up easily. He prescribed me an oral form on the infusion to bridge the transition between hospital and home as well as insisting I do a pain management program. I felt I was cured when I left the hospital yet he said that I had a long way to go. In hindsight he was right because really that was just the beginning of me getting better. It wasn't until I took part in that pain management program that I started to take control and learnt to manage the pain.

Prior to being put into this pain management program, the idea that what you do rather than what you take has more to do with pain control had been raised with me by several close friends. One an anaesthetist, the other a physiotherapist both suggested I should try meditation and relaxation, but it just seemed like hippie stuff and I said that it wouldn't work for my migraines because they were real, not in my head. They knew the way I would finally get through this was to realise the relationship between my mind and my migraines but that I was probably only going to understand that relationship when I was ready. At the time I didn't understand that - when you are so in the thick of it and you are surrounded by medications and you can just take a pill. It is so hard to actually think that you can change this. I couldn't even contemplate making a change like that.

Both Prof and my doctor insisted I do this pain management program. On the morning going out there I thought that it was going to be a waste of time. When I walked into the room all I could see was a whole lot of people in pain. I didn't think that I could relate to any of them. They all told similar stories of living on drugs and being trapped inside their body with pain. I didn't want to view myself as "one of them" but my story was very similar. There was only myself and one other person in the room who had someone to care and support them - I thought that was devastating.

Once the instructors started talking about pain I was enthralled. I'd never heard anything like what I was hearing about how pain worked and the worst thing was that I was a biology lecturer - I didn't understand pain at all. I thought that this was outrageous. I had lived with pain all my life and no one had ever explained pain to me. I was sitting there feeling angry and embarrassed and almost in tears - I was completely overwhelmed. I felt like it was a complete waste of my life and I had needed to know about all of this years ago. Even though they weren't specifically talking about migraines it all made sense to me and I could see how it could apply to me.

The techniques that I took away from that were honestly the things that have made the biggest difference in my life. I have reduced the amount of medication that I am on. Despite often waking up with a headache, I now know I have to get out of bed regardless because nine times out of ten I always feel better. I try and take that positive attitude with me as I face the day ahead and usually find my pain is unnoticed within an hour or so. If I start to feel angry or stressed my pain level can increase very quickly. I've learnt to be able to control that anger or those feelings and subsequently reduce the pain. I've also recognised that keeping busy and distracted is the best pain relief of all. Getting back to work was really important for me - it gave me some purpose and kept me busy. I found that 95% of the time I was able to avoid a migraine or keep it at bay. It doesn't always work but now I can go for months without a migraine. Also, now when I do get a migraine, I don't panic because I know that I can get through it without medication. I can wake up now with a migraine where I feel so bad and so sick but I know that the chances are that I will get through this because I have before. I don't identify with being a person who has migraines that rule my life anymore and the best thing is that I get to put my boys to bed every night.

SAMIA

I have always been an active person. Growing up I rode my bike everywhere and played a number of different sports. At the time of my knee injury I was playing tennis, soccer, netball and dancing. I tried physiotherapy for weeks but it wasn't improving so I was referred to an orthopaedic surgeon who said I needed an arthroscope. The MRI showed the fat pad in my knee needed to be shaved back as it had worn down from overuse. I was 25 at the time, I hadn't done anything in particular to trigger the pain. It wasn't the result of a sports injury or from my dancing, it was just playing up and I knew it wasn't right. My surgeon explained it was a minor operation and I would be back to normal activities in eight to twelve weeks.

The operation was in May 2007 and it went well. The surgeon removed part of the antero medical retro-patella fat pad which appeared to be impinging and causing pain and swelling. Otherwise the knee appeared in excellent condition. I woke up and I started rehabilitation immediately. I was on crutches for only a day or two and then started walking again. I was vigilant in doing all the exercises the physiotherapist prescribed and things were going really well. Then one day, four weeks after the surgery, I was getting off the tram and couldn't walk 100 metres across the road to my boyfriend's house. My knee just stopped working and I wasn't able to stand on it.

Naturally, I was really worried because it had been going so well and then all of a sudden it wasn't working at all. I rang my surgeon and unfortunately he was on leave so I had to wait a very long eight weeks before I could see him. I couldn't walk at all, I had no choice but to call my parents and get the crutches back out of the garage. I was devastated.

During this awful wait to see the surgeon, not knowing what was wrong, my knee was experiencing colour changes. It would go dark blue and then change to red. I was experiencing strange sensations in my knee, it would go hot and cold, I would get sharp stabbing pains and constant burning sensations. My leg had also wasted away and my jeans were really loose around my thigh.

When I finally got to see my surgeon he sent me off to get an MRI to see what had gone wrong. More waiting. It was another few weeks before I got the results. My surgeon reviewed the MRI and examined my knee. He said there was nothing structurally wrong with it. He suspected I may have a nerve condition, but felt he had done his "part' and referred me to a pain specialist.

It was a waiting game again, another month until I got in to see the pain specialist. The waiting is the worst part; the unknown. Your mind thinks the worst during this time. In August 2007, approximately four months after my operation, I saw the pain specialist for the first time. He diagnosed me with having Reflex Sympathetic Dystrophy (RSD) which later became known as Complex Regional Pain Syndrome (CRPS). He said patients who suffer from fibromyalgia also have a higher chance of getting this condition. I was diagnosed with fibromyalgia when I was 19. While my fibromyalgia was very debilitating in the first few years, I knew its trigger signs and had managed it reasonably well since, so it came as a surprise to hear the condition gave me a higher chance of getting CRPS.

I felt like the specialist was very vague. Each consult lasted five minutes and he would just do the standard sensory testing on my leg with the tissue and then prescribe me a different drug or alter my existing dose of drugs. I didn't feel like he listened to me, avoided my questions and there was never a clear treatment pathway or definitive answers. I wanted to know if I was ever going to walk again and he wasn't able to give me any indication.

I asked him how other people get this condition and he explained from gunshot wounds, snake bites, or after major surgeries as a result of the trauma. I found the information really alarming, how could I have the same condition as someone who had been shot?

You go to see a specialist with the expectation they will conduct a thorough assessment and discuss a treatment plan. I was furious and upset each time I left his rooms, spending money yet never getting a clear pathway forward.

I persisted with this trial and error approach for about a year, which involved three phentolamine infusions and a daily cocktail of drugs. While some days I thought it was helping, other days I felt I was back to where I started. The side effects were becoming just as difficult to deal with as the condition itself. Since I wasn't improving, I felt like I had lost a whole part of my life. I was having a really tough time at work, travelling to and from the office on crutches and experiencing a lot of pain. My manager and colleagues didn't understand the condition and it was hard to describe it to them.

My manager was very unsupportive and I was worried I was going to get fired. My pain specialists advised I needed to work three days a week from home to see if resting my knee more would aid my recovery. I was seeing the physiotherapist and trying to do everything she suggested but it felt like I was fighting a losing battle and going around in circles.

I got to a point where I had enough of being on medication and the side effects that went with them. I felt if I stayed on the same path I would be having the same conversations with the pain specialist in 40 years' time!

He would keep getting out his script book and be prescribing me drugs. I'd be in that waiting room, no better. I knew the body has amazing capabilities and I'd enjoyed training and keeping fit all my life. I wanted to do more to help myself. So in September 2007 I starting working a lot harder in the pool. I was there every morning at 6am with the seniors doing my exercises. It helped having the regulars there; you felt like part of a community. Being in the pool your body is weightless, so for a glimpse I would feel better. I just focussed on the exercise program my physiotherapist gave me and followed it each day.

Around this time, a trip to Turkey I had booked with a friend was approaching. I was really excited and wanted to go but I was hesitant because I didn't want to burden my friend. I didn't want to hold her back as I still wasn't able to walk properly. I love to travel and I love exploring places on foot, I think it's the best way to see a city. Sadly I knew this trip wouldn't be like that. My friend was incredibly understanding and said we would work around it, get taxis if we needed to. I went on the trip and was determined to see as much as I could!

On one of our excursions, we did a walk which had a steep descent and I wasn't sure how I was going to tackle it. There was a physiotherapist in our tour group and she said, just try going down Sarah, even if you have to shuffle down on your backside, just give it a go. And that is exactly what I did!

I am not sure if it was sliding down that hill that fired the muscles in my legs, or being more active on the trip in general (probably a combination of both), but the very next day I will remember forever. I was walking up the steps of our accommodation, both feet on the step, the only way I had been able to tackle stairs for the last six months, but this time I pushed myself a little harder. I put my sore leg on the step and forced some weight through it, and for the first time in six months it worked! It actually took my weight. I will never ever forget that moment. Up until then, I really never knew if I would walk again.

My trip to Turkey and being able to put weight through my leg filled me with hope. When I returned home I was even more determined with my exercises in the pool and eventually progressed to the gym.

I started being able to walk without any aids and gradually grew stronger. My physiotherapist continued to be an enormous help and ongoing support for me. She would prescribe exercises each visit and taught me the important lesson of taking it slowly. My nature was when I saw a little bit of improvement, it would give me hope and then I would push myself really hard. I would end up in pain and then I would get terrified it would go backwards and I would end up where I started. She taught me how to do my exercises in small increments at the gym. For instance, starting with 30 seconds on the cross trainer, building it up gradually to one minute, then one and a half minutes and so on. Having usually gone to the gym for an hour and working out hard and leaving exhausted, I found this so annoying and embarrassing to turn up and go on a machine for 30 seconds! So it took me a while to come around, but I eventually realised she was right and now I understand and listen to my body a lot more.

It took about two more years of gradual training before things got better in the middle of 2009. The pain and the colour changes as well as the burning and hot and cold sensations hung around for a long time but finally they went away. I had a few good years when things were okay and life was close to being back to normal. I wasn't able to return to sport which has always been upsetting but I have come to accept that now. I look at what I am able to do and I am grateful. My pain specialist said if I return to sport there was a risk I could get injured and the CRPS would likely flair up and I may not be able to walk again. His words have always rung in my ears. My grandparents have always been a very inspiring influence in guiding my thoughts. My Nanna would say "Oh well, if you can't play tennis, find another hobby to do.'

Things had been going along well for a few years and then in 2012 I began training for a hike in Italy with my sister. I increased my training a lot over the following year and noticed my hip starting to get sore. It started with a niggling pain and it would come and go. I tried physiotherapy for a while and then I realised it was a real problem and I went and got an MRI. The results showed I had a congenitally shallow hip joint which was causing the trouble. I went back to my original orthopaedic surgeon who explained it would need surgery. He was very aware of my history and talked it through thoroughly with me. He made me aware that there was a chance the CRPS could come back again if we went ahead with surgery. He said because I was young and active it was likely it would need to be done, especially if it was interfering with my life. However, ultimately it was my decision to make. I decided to wait and really think about what I wanted to do. It had taken me so long to get over CRPS the last time, I dreaded the thought of having another operation and having to go through the whole ordeal again.

The next 18 months were extremely challenging for me physically, mentally and emotionally. I didn't want to have the surgery and I was hoping my hip would correct itself. Being active is part of who I am, when my hip got sore I couldn't exercise the way I had been, which was already limited from having CRPS, and as a result I felt so down. Then the day to day activities became harder, sitting for a full day of work, walking around on a weekend, standing to cook dinner, bending over to clean the bathroom, carrying in the shopping. Simple tasks, but they all became a struggle. Gone were the days I could wear heels. I lived in runners for the better part of two years and didn't feel good about myself.

My boyfriend at the time was so incredibly supportive, he would help in every way possible. He listened to me
when I was down, came to appointments with me, drove
me around when I couldn't, did the grocery shopping,
cooked for us, cleaned the house, the list goes on. He was
there for me day in and day out. And yet while he did all
these things to help, I just felt guilty, like I wasn't able to
contribute to the relationship. We had recently moved in
together when all this flared up and I felt useless and like
I was no fun to be around at all.

My boyfriend and I went on a trip to Portugal the
following year in July 2014. We had been walking around
Lisbon all day and we had one more sight at the top of the
hill we wanted to see. But I couldn't walk another step. I
said to my boyfriend, you go ahead, I will meet you back
at the apartment. I knew then that I couldn't' go on like
this. Yes the risk was there I would get CRPS again, 20%
chance I recall, but I couldn't go on the way I was.

Obviously, I was really nervous about getting the
surgery done, which probably didn't help matters.
I had the procedure in February 2015 on my left hip,
the opposite side to my earlier knee injury. I had a
pincer impingement with early labral degeneration and
chondrolabral separation. He took down the laburm,
removed approximately 4mm of rim bone along with
areas of acute calcification, and then repaired the
labrum with anchors and sutures.

I was in a lot of pain afterwards. I ended up getting CRPS again. It was traumatic to go through it all again but this time I knew what was happening and people around understood as well. I went through all the rehabilitation again, mainly driven by that same determination and knowing I had recovered once before. Work was really challenging again. My manager at the time made my life really difficult and I am sure this added stress didn't help my recovery. Nobody in my new job really understood because I would have good days and bad days and this time I wasn't on crutches so people couldn't see something was wrong. It gradually got better as I got back to exercise and the pain went away.

Later the same year, as I was getting better, my other hip started playing up. I couldn't believe it! It was a congenital problem and my sister had needed her hip done when she was 17 so there was probably also a genetic component. I had the scan and the surgeon said it needed to be operated on. This time I was really pro-active. I didn't wait until it got really bad which I think helped as the surgery wasn't as major or traumatic. The surgeon was well aware of my history and explained he would do what he could to minimise the trauma during the operation. I also contacted the anaesthetist prior to the surgery. We discussed my history and he outlined several options available to me. This put me at ease immensely, it gave me a sense of relief and comfort knowing the anaesthetist understood my history and was going to take extra precautions to minimise the pain prior, during and post operation.

I had the operation on my right hip in October 2015. I had a pincer impingement with minor labral damage and partial thickness ligamentum teres tear. My surgeon was able to remove the excessive acetabular rim bone from behind the labrum without having to detach the labrum. This meant that they didn't have to insert anchors and sutures to repair the labrum after rim trimming. As a rule this leads to a faster and smoother recovery.

I didn't get CRPS again, thank goodness! I think the combination of the surgery not being as complex, the surgeon taking precautions to cause less damage and having the support of the anaesthetist monitoring my pain relief throughout the operation made the difference.

By the following June 2016, when I was back to full health, I resigned from my job and went traveling. I climbed volcanoes in Nicaragua, went hiking in the jungle in Belize, sky dived in South Africa, scaled mountains in Colombia and played soccer with the locals in Guatemala. I was on the road for almost two years. My body has never been as good as it was during that time. I was relaxed and having the time of my life! I don't think we are designed to be sitting at a desk all day. I believe we are designed to move.

I have been home only a few months now and still

going strong. I have my ups and downs like everyone else and I still battle with trying to find the balance of keeping active but not over doing it. I will always have the desire to train hard, but I have learnt over the years to listen to my body and I am so grateful when it works in harmony. I am happiest now when I find a balance and my body functions normally to get through a day's activities.

I have recently started a mindfulness workshop and I am so proud to say I have made it to 45 minutes of mindfulness body scans five days in a row! A miracle for me. Exercising and being active I find easy, my real challenge is learning how to work through the pain when it's at its worst. Once the cycle starts it is hard to stop it.

I am excited about the mindfulness practice and what it can offer when I am in pain. Combine that with my regular exercise and I think I'll have a winning combination. There is a reason my body felt better than ever while I was travelling and I want to tap into how to replicate that back home.

My advice to anyone reading this book who has CRPS, is to not give up first and foremost. Don't be afraid of the pain, keep persisting, see different health professionals and specialists, and try new ways of exercising and strengthening the muscles. I am so thankful I persisted. Once I broke the cycle of pain and got my muscles moving, great things came as a result.

Surrounding yourself with a good support system

- family, friends and health professionals, I think is a key part of surviving and living with this condition. I also learnt not talking about my pain helped. It's natural to want to talk about it, vent your frustrations to your closest ones. However in the end, I think with everyone asking me how my hip was, my knee or my other hip, it would always bring it back to the forefront of my mind, draw my attention to it again and again. And it may have been the one time I wasn't thinking about it!

Lastly, to recognise pain specialists will treat CRPS in a trial and error approach. As each patient suffers differently, the specialist will try different methods to see what works best. In hindsight I wish the specialist had explained this more clearly to me. I think it would have helped me manage the condition better and reduce my stress levels throughout the entire process.

Thank you Alison for asking me to share my story and to my parents for their endless love and support. I hope it helps others suffering with CRPS and gives them a sense of hope that there can be light at the end of the tunnel!!

UNDERSTANDING PAIN

Reading these incredibly personal, difficult and sometimes heartbreaking stories gives us an up close and
personal understanding of how pain can interfere with
a person's life. It helps us to put ourselves in their shoes
and understand, if only to a small extent, the suffering
that people with persistent pain experience. It invades all
facets of life, stripping away the good bits, taking away
the parts that define who we are. It leaves behind a life
of medical appointments, conflicting diagnoses, uncertainty about the future, money worries and ultimately
fear – that the pain will get worse, that you may not be
able to cope, that you will never be "you" again.

The hopeful theme in all these stories however, is that
all of the people interviewed experienced a turning point
in their journey and after that, things started to improve.
Many of them got to a point where they could say "pain
just isn't a thing for me any more". They may still experience pain, but it no longer controls every part of their life.
In this section of the book, I am hoping to describe to you

elements of what it was that helped these people to turn the corner and begin to get back to life. The underpinning ideas in this approach that these people have used, is largely based on a modern, science based understanding of pain and the nervous system. One that moves away from quick fixes, magic silver bullets and miracle cures and embraces what we know about the science of pain.

You might have noticed that many of people's situation improved once they learned about pain. Some clinicians describe this as pain education or therapeutic neuroscience education, others call it explaining pain. The long and short of this approach is the idea that once we better understand the nature of pain – the nuts and bolts, the physiology and the nervous system, pain becomes less mysterious. When it is less of a mystery and we can better understand how to reverse some of the changes that have occurred, suddenly we can feel like there is a way out of the pain hole. The message is incredibly self empowering – we can play a massive role in making that happen for ourselves. We don't have to wait for it to be done to us by someone else or something else. We understand what we were already starting to realise as we chased the medical appointments and the various treatments aimed to reduce our pain – there is no quick fix.

You might also notice that many of the people interviewed had some doubts about whether this approach would work for them. When we have been convinced for so long that the answer or cure is out there and we just need to find the right practitioner, the right modality, the right intervention to take it all away, giving up on that merry-go-round can be an upsetting process. My hope is that these stories can help people who are stuck on the merry-go-round see that these approaches can work really well at getting you back to doing the things that are important – the things that pain may have taken away.

Your pain experience

As you have probably seen from the stories and will further learn when we explore pain science, pain can be an incredibly invisible illness. Many times there is nothing to see on an x-ray or MRI, injuries that might have started a process have well and truly healed or there may be no explanation or diagnosis at all for the pain. Other times, something might be seen on an MRI, but we know that lots of people have those same changes and don't experience pain. This is incredibly frustrating because despite not having many answers, the pain is real. The pain is very real. It is distressing, it is upsetting and it interferes with life. However because it is often invisible, friends, work colleagues and family may find it hard to understand. Many people report being told "you don't look sick" or "it can't be that bad". Other people have experiences of frustration, anger or shame after seeing medical and health professionals who seem to not believe their story, dismiss their concerns or offer no helpful solutions. It can be easy for a person with pain to feel like others believe they are faking, malingering or just haven't tried hard enough to get better. This can lead to feelings of such helplessness and sadness, unhelpful emotions for someone trying to get out of a pain problem.

THE SCIENCE

So what is this science that explains why pain hangs around longer than it should in some people?

Firstly, it's important to understand how pain works in the normal setting.

Acute pain

Acute or short term pain usually comes on when there has been tissue damage. Nerves in the tissues that specifically carry information about inflammation, mechanical damage and high thermal information, are activated when something has gone wrong with the tissues. For example a joint sprain, intervertebral disc damage, muscle strain or bone fracture. The nerves in the tissues that carry the information about this, send the messages to the spinal cord and into the brain. At the same time, the chemicals created in the inflammation associated with the damage, sensitise nerves in the surrounding area and make it easier for them to send a signal. In other words, their threshold for sending a signal becomes significantly lower. We could describe them as being a bit jumpy and on the look out for other damage.

That information travels up the spinal cord and into the brain. It arrives at a lower area of the brain known as the thalamus, which is sometimes described as a relay station. From this area, the signals are directed to a variety of areas in the brain which are known to be active in the presence of pain. (We know this because scientists have demonstrated that these areas consistently become active when we expose healthy people to experimental pain situations and measure their brain activity using a functional MRI.)

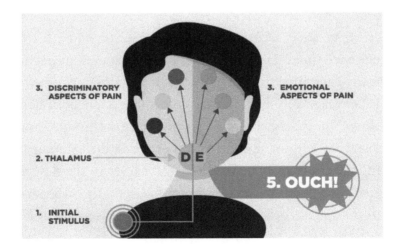

Some areas of the thalamus (relay station) are associated with delegating information about the more discriminatory aspects of the information. They help the brain to get an understanding of where the damage is, what type of sensation it is, how large is the affected area and other more tangible aspects of the situation. This helps the brain to start to create a picture about how much of a big deal the situation is.

The other components of the signals in the thalamus are relayed to areas of the brain that are known to be associated with more emotional circuitry. This is an important survival mechanism for us because without having an emotional reaction to tissue damage, it is unlikely that we would change our behaviour. Without changing our behaviour we might keep doing the same things again and continue to damage our tissues. So engaging the emotional circuitry is a clever way of making us pay attention, stop the damaging processes and protect the damaged area. Fear is a great motivator in these situations and the areas of the brain that are known to be very active in fear situations, tend to light up consistently in pain situations. Memory and social understandings of pain can also play a role in these more emotional components of a pain experience. Areas of the brain that store memories about previous pain experiences may be activated and will contribute to the picture that the brain creates. Additionally, contextual clues about the situation from other areas of the brain will add information, for example about how society views that particular situation or if other people you know might have had similar experiences.

With both the discriminatory and the emotional aspects of the information being processed by the brain, together with information from vision and hearing systems, the context of the situation and memories of previous pain experiences, the brain puts together a story about the information. If the story is one where the brain believes that there is danger or that the collective information has a lot of meaning, it will create pain. Pain is designed in this instance to make us pay attention and change our behaviour. If we think about it from a "survival of the species" point of view, without pain, we would be less likely to change our behaviour in the presence of tissue damage, would be more likely to create further damage and would reduce the likelihood of the species continuing to thrive. Pain is designed to help us survive.

Straight away, we can see that what has gone on in the tissue does not equally equate to a level of pain that experienced. The big mediating factor is the brain and all of the contextual information that is stored within it. If those incoming nerve signals from the body are interpreted by the brain to have a lot of meaning, pain is a likely outcome. However if the brain puts together all the information and context and decides that the nerve signals do not represent a threat, it may decide not to create pain.

We see examples of this on both sides of the spectrum. There have been amazing cases in the medical field where people have experienced significant tissue damage but present with little or not pain. Examples of this might include fight sports where a painless but clearly broken nose received in the process of winning a gold medal is viewed as positive or a normal part of the sport. Other examples include a person who lost a limb in a car accident and needed to escape from a burning car, only to realise much later that the limb was lost. In this instance his brain had decided that pain was not a priority compared to escaping the burning car.

On the flip side there have been examples of people experiencing extreme pain following assumed tissue damage such as the poor fellow who thought he had impaled himself in the foot with a nail gun. The case study, published in the British Medical Journal, describes the story of a man who presented to the emergency department with a nail through his boot, appearing to go through his foot. He was distressed and in considerable pain and required sedation and pain relief. When it came to removing the nail, doctors discover the nail had landed happily between his toes and not created any tissue damage. The visual context provided to his brain of the image of his foot with a nail in it, together with the knowledge that this was a big deal and that a nail in the foot would cause damage, meant that his brain created an output of pain to make him do something about the situation – in this case to present himself to the emergency department. It is important at this point to recognise that the pain the person is experiencing is real, despite the lack of tissue damage – this is how clever our pain systems are!

The messages that we receive from the people around us can play a big role in how our brain interprets the situation and therefore the level of pain that it will create as an output. Consider a situation where a child falls over and skins his knee and looks immediately towards Mum. When mum responds by calmly reassuring the child, applying "placebo" kisses to the knee, and encouraging them to quickly return to their play, the child will invariably feel less pain and distress. If Mum was to look worried, cry out, and make a catastrophic fuss about the skinned knee, the child is way more likely to feel more pain and distress about the situation, because his brain has taken into consideration that Mum is worried and therefore, maybe so should he.

The parallel situation exists frequently in our medical systems. We are given many and varied messages by health care practitioners, friends and family and the media about our ailments. Worrying messages received about MRI reports like "its bone on bone" or "there are two big disc bulges" can change the way we view our body, making us more worried, fearful of creating more damage and worried about moving. Social cues coming from well meaning work colleagues that caution about ending up "like Fred in the wheelchair whose problems started just like yours" can have subconscious influence. Similarly cultural and family expectations about pain can influence our own pain experiences. "You have your grandfather's back" or "its in our genes" can be powerful messages that influence how our brain interprets those messages from the tissues.

Our science is starting to paint us some very clear pictures about these long held but largely unhelpful beliefs about the body and about pain. We now understand very well that what we see on an x-ray or MRI does not correlate well at all with pain levels. Many people with no pain at all have extensive osteoarthritis changes in their joints and similarly, most people over the age of 40 have at least one disc bulge in their back, the vast majority of which are not painful at all. We are starting to view these imaging findings as incidental and some are describing them as wrinkles on the inside – they don't look pretty but they don't hurt! In my own practice I recently saw a young and fit male who was sent for an MRI for a leg problem and happened to have his back scanned in the process. The scan discovered a disc bulge in his low back, one that had likely been sitting there for years without causing problems. The way that these results were conveyed to him created worry about his previously pain free back. Within days he developed back pain and for three years suffered with disabling, distressing pain. With some reassurance and education about his condition he recovered very well, very quickly, but I couldn't help thinking about what a waste those three years were for him and how he could have done without all of that distress. Whilst MRIs and other imaging techniques have an important role to play in picking up serious pathology, their high sensitivity means that they pick up things that otherwise would have not been seen and may never have been a problem. There is a strong understanding in the medical and pain community about this phenomenon of over-imaging and how unhelpful it can be for many people.

Back at the level of those nerves in our initially damaged tissues, as the damage heals and the inflammation resides, the messages to the spinal cord and brain from that area should also reduce or stop. The damaged areas may scar in the healing process and the area may end up stronger than it was before, if perhaps a little less mobile. Ultimately, at this point in time, the area is safe and healed. Further damage is unlikely and normal function can be restored on a gradual basis. Depending on what tissue was initially involved and how extensive the damage was, this process can take weeks or months to occur. Generally, most tissues will have largely healed within three months and the tissues are safe and sound. It is understandable at this time that people may feel hesitant to return to using that body part, especially if they are worried that it may become damaged again. But its important to realise that tissues generally heal well and using them in a gradual way helps the healing and strengthening process.

In some instances, despite the fact that the tissues have healed, the pain still hangs around. In these cases, the pain is real, however it doesn't tell a very true picture of what is happening in the tissue, compared to how it did when it first started.

Changes occur in the nervous system that can help to explain why this pain hangs around longer than it should. Firstly, in the brain, when there are many worrisome thoughts about the pain and the condition, those areas of the brain that are associated with the emotional aspects, can become more and more active. This makes sense – pain is not pleasant and there can be lots of things to worry about – is this going to get worse? Am I going to get better? Am I going to lose my job because of this? What if I can't take care of my kids? How will I ever get back to the things that I enjoy doing? What if I end up like Aunt Mary in a wheelchair? The doctor said that my MRI results were terrible.

When these areas become really active they can have

an influence on our Fight, Flight and Fright systems (sympathetic nervous system) which tends to up-regulate our stress hormones. These systems and hormones are supposed to work in the short term – in short bursts throughout the day. However when we are constantly worried about our pain and what it means, they can become overactive and constantly switched on. This has the effect of bathing our body in stress hormones, including the original area that was affected. These hormones and chemicals affect the nerves by continually sensitising them so that they don't need much input from the tissues to send a message to the brain. In fact, these nerves can become so sensitised and jumpy that it doesn't even need a stimulus to send a signal – it can just send them for the sake of it. This means that even though the tissue may have healed well and is getting back to being strong and healthy, there is still input coming from the area telling the brain that all is not well.

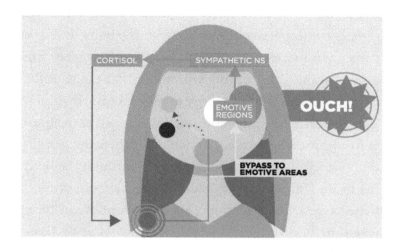

As time progresses and the emotional circuitry of the brain stays active because the worries about the pain continue, those discriminatory areas of the brain that told us where, what and how much about the tissue damage tend to be less active. They almost become a bit neglected. So whilst we are still experiencing pain, the areas that are supposed to tell that very true picture about the tissues are essentially silent. The take home point from these changes is that whilst the pain is very real, it is not telling a very true picture about what is going on at the level of the tissue.

Another factor that plays into our experience of pain is the fact that we have very good internal pain relieving systems. When things are relaxed, this system is designed to be on and to act as a filter. Messages that originate from specific areas of the brain send signals down the spinal cord. These signals are designed to stop signals coming up to the brain from the body. It blocks the signals because the brain is not in an alert state and doesn't want to be dealing with all of that excess information. It takes a lot of energy to process information so it keeps this filter system on as a default. When the brain is in a more alert state, particularly when those fight, flight or fright chemicals are surging through the body, the brain will tend to switch off these filters in order to better assess the situation. This is appropriate in times when the brain needs to get a good idea of acute tissue damage. However, in persistent pain, the tissue damage has healed but the worrisome thoughts, and hence the stress chemicals are still surging around the body and brain. This means that this filter system is constantly being prompted to switch off and therefore the brain is getting far more information than it needs. Most of this information would normally be below a threshold that the brain would pay attention to. The brain is bombarded with information that ordinarily wouldn't make it through and suddenly things that shouldn't hurt, start to hurt. This is where our pain can spread to other body parts and aches and pains that we could normally ignore suddenly become a big deal.

Knowing that these things are occurring in our nervous system often helps people to really understand certain facets about their pain. Why, for example, does the pain often come and go for no real reason? Why does it get worse when I get stressed out? It can also be really helpful to understand that feeling pain does not mean that there is tissue damage. In the context of starting to move more and get the area stronger and more capable, this message can be a game changer. These messages that the tissues are safe and healed and that the pain doesn't have as much meaning can be reassuring enough in some cases to reduce that overactivity in the emotional circuitry in the brain and reduce the distress that often goes hand in hand with pain.

So we now understand that whilst the pain is very real and very distressing, it doesn't mean that it is coming from tissue damage. We could view the situation better by saying that the problem now lies with the nervous system and no longer in the tissues where the initial problem was. The good thing is, most of these changes are completely reversible. It has changed one way and it can change back. This process is known as neuroplasticity.

In order to get those more discriminatory areas of the brain to pay better attention to the effected region and recognise that good healing has occurred and that everything is okay, the effected body part needs to be used the way that it is designed to be used. Doing this in a repeated and useful way that replicates doing the things that you have been avoiding helps to re-wire those neglected areas. It is effectively like taking a more accurate snapshot of the tissues and reporting back on a more updated and ultimately safe situation.

The paradox with this is that movement is often the thing that makes pain worse and so this idea can seem completely counter intuitive. Reflecting back on the idea that the pain doesn't represent tissue damage can be really helpful in embracing this idea. If pain doesn't mean that damage is being done, then experiencing a bit of pain in the process of getting better is okay. The key to this idea is just how much pain is okay to experience when using a movement approach and how to grade and implement these movement approaches. Fortunately, these days we know a lot about this and there are some good concepts that can help to guide you.

Pacing or Graded Exposure

The process of introducing movement rehabilitation for chronic pain is known as a few different things. Sometimes it is called pacing, other people might call it graded exposure or graded exercise. Essentially they are the same thing. The basic idea is that in order to work towards doing something that you haven't been able to do, you start very slowly and build up using fairly strictly prescribed increments to increase the movement. This means that your nervous system and tissues are exposed to the movement gradually and it can take its time to adapt. An example might be that if you wanted to be able to get back to bike riding but you found that going for a 30 minute ride gave you a lot of pain for several days after the bike ride, you might set a graded exposure approach that looked like this:

Day 1: 2 minutes slow riding
Day 2: 3 minutes slow riding
Day 3: 5 minutes slow riding
Day 4: 5 minutes slow – medium pace
Day 5: 7 minutes slow – medium pace
Day 6: 10 minutes slow pace
Day 7: 10 minutes slow – medium pace

Week 2
Gradually building to 20 minutes slow pace

Week 3
Gradually building to 20 minutes slow – medium pace

Week 4
Gradually building to 30 minutes slow pace

Week 5
Gradually building to 30 minutes slow – medium pace

This is just an example and many factors would dictate

how fast or slow you progress the exercises, but some of the principles that we stick to are:

1. Start low and go slow – even if it seems silly. A sensitive nervous system will appreciate it.
2. Stick with the prescribed increments. Don't do more even if you are feeling good.
3. If you have increased pain the next day or after doing the exercise, don't panic – remember that it doesn't mean that you have done damage, just that you have hit that flare up line (see below). Know that it will pass and that you can get back to the program quickly. Many people suggest that rather than doing nothing at all at these times, that you do half of the prescribed amount or less for a few days and then try to get back to the point of the program that you were at.
4. If you have had a flare up or two you might like to consider slowing the incremental raises – most practitioners would suggest that you halve the size of the increments.

The best thing about this approach is that you can apply it to almost anything that you would like to get back to doing. Its also the approach that we use when we are doing gym based exercise rehabilitation programs. You can adjust the increments by using the number of repetitions, the time spent exercising, the intensity of the exercise (you could measure this with heart rate monitoring), the amount of weight or resistance. It also doesn't have to be a specific exercise, it can be anything that you would like to get back to doing. If gardening is something that you really loved and wanted to do, you might start with one to two minutes of weeding and gradually increase the time you spend in the garden. If it was playing with the grandkids on the floor, you might start with just reading a short book on the floor and then move to slightly more vigorous activities another day.

The most important idea of this approach is that you do enough to expose the nervous and muscular systems to the movement so that they make adjustments in response to it, but not enough to cause pain on a regular basis. It is normal to have some times of increased pain, especially when we are starting activities that we aren't used to, but we don't want to be working so hard each time to be causing dramatic increases in pain on a regular basis. Its meant to be a slow and steady process and requires a lot of discipline and patience.

I use these diagrams to help people to understand the concept a bit more. In this first chart, it shows the idea that in a healthy body, we have the capacity to actually cause ourselves damage by over doing things – whether by an accident that causes strain or damage to tissues, or just by physically over exerting ourselves. Usually though, our nervous system protects us from getting to that point by creating pain when we are nearing that level. I have called that the flare up line in this diagram and you can see that it leaves a buffer of space below the point where damage will actually occur. It acts like a proximity alarm when we get close to or actually hit the damage line.

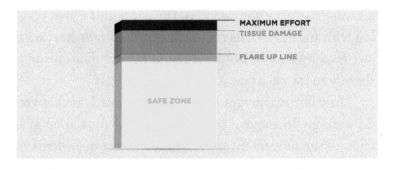

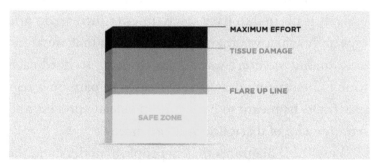

This second diagram represents a nervous system that is sensitised – like one that has persistent pain. You can see that the flare up line has been artificially lowered by the sensitisation process. It sits well below the point where damage is going to occur. Essentially, you have less capacity below the line so it is easy to hit the flare up line. Also when you do hit it, you were not at all close to doing damage to your tissues. I liken this to a car alarm that goes off when someone enters the garage, rather than when someone is actually trying to break into the car. It doesn't really tell us a true picture of what is going on.

In a graded exposure or pacing approach, we need to work under the flare up line in the safe zone, but close enough to it so that we actually expose the tissue to movement so that it can adapt. Sometimes we end up inadvertently hitting the flare up line in order to find out where it is. This is not a big deal and sometimes we could even view this as being helpful. It allows us to know what our limits are so that we can work just underneath that.

Over time as we work underneath that flare up line and the tissues are being exposed to movement that is safe, comfortable and not always painful, the flare up line can start to move up to a place that represents what is actually going on in the tissues a bit more accurately. This means that as our tissues become more resilient, we experience less flare ups and have a greater capacity to do more things.

When we take the fear out of flare up, we are more likely to give movement or exercise a go because we are not worried that we are causing damage or going backwards. Knowing that it is largely due to the sensitisation of the system, that it will pass on its own and that it doesn't mean too much can be a really powerful concept to hold onto when we have some pain after exercise.

During a flare up, as well as reassuring ourselves that everything is okay and that it will go away with time, there are also some things that we can try to help get through it. These might include using heat packs, cold packs, gentle stretching, mindfulness relaxation, TENs machines, topical creams, gentle massage or foam rolling. Sometimes medication approaches might be appropriate in these instances too if you know that it is just a stop gap to help get you through. Whilst these are unlikely to completely take the pain away and they are not all appropriate to do all the time, during a flare up they may just be able to reduce the pain levels a bit to make it more bearable while it passes. Then we can get back to the pacing program sooner and keep making progress.

Many people find the idea of movement or exercise programs in the presence of pain very confronting. It can be hard to really embrace the idea that it isn't going to cause damage, especially if those beliefs have been held for a long time, or a care giver has specifically told you to avoid certain movement. While those cautions may have been appropriate early in the healing process, when using a slow and steady approach like this, it is rare that specific movements will need to be avoided in the long term. It can be really helpful to have someone who is trained in this approach to help you with the process. They can help you to discover ways of moving without it hurting so much, encourage you to persist when you are feeling uncertain and hold you back when you are overdoing it. Exercise rehabilitation has the largest body of evidence when it comes to looking at what works in getting people back to function with persistent pain. Trying an approach like this and giving up because you either had too much pain or didn't make enough progress can be really unhelpful because it can lead you to believe that exercise doesn't help for your particular condition. Having someone there to guide you can help stop this from happening and encourage good progress.

Adopting an active approach in getting back to being you can be the most important step in recovery, and I think that the stories that were told by our pain heroes quite consistently demonstrated this. An active approach simply means that you are trying to do something to help yourself, rather than waiting for someone or something else to do it for you. The opposite to this is passive approaches. Those are the ones where you are having something done to you, waiting for someone else to find a cure, or something to just take the pain away for you. Whilst these are appealing ideas, and many miracle cures and therapy modalities are sold to very vulnerable people based on these ideas, the reality is that these approaches don't work in persistent pain. Having an active mindset and knowing that you can help yourself are very important to help take back control of your situation. You may have noticed that many of the pain heroes reported a sensation of feeling lost or out of control in their pain journey. The consistent messages from their stories were that once people understood more about what pain was, and importantly what pain wasn't, they were better able to adopt approaches that were aimed at helping themselves. They changed their mindsets and began to apply pacing principles to getting back to their lives. This active versus passive concept is truly a big part of turning the pain story around. It is also backed by large amounts of research that tells us that active approaches are consistently more effective for treating persistent pain, compared to passive approaches.

Pain is an all encompassing experience and many people find that once it has hung around for a long time, life revolves around it. This means that all the good bits – the bits of life that make us happy, engaged and enjoy life, fall by the wayside. Part of an active approach might be to start to expand the good bits of life that have been forgotten.

This diagram gives us the idea that when pain is present, life around it becomes small and usually revolves around seeking medical appointments, focusing on wanting our pain to go away and avoiding things that we think are going to hurt.

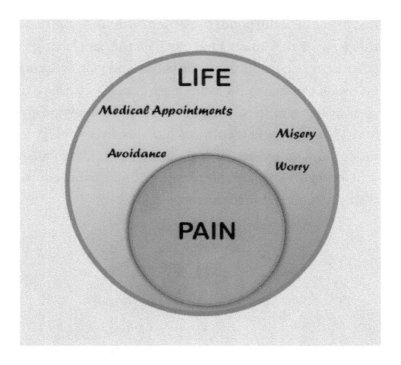

We tend to focus on looking at things that will shrink the pain, and there are some things that can be helpful in doing that, although they take a long time and take some persistent effort. However, sometimes another way to look at the situation is to review some of the good things that pain has taken away from us, and start to get back to doing those. These are usually things that align with the idea that we are living a life that fits with our values. For example we might like to get back to watching live music gigs, traveling, photography, spending time with friends or family, playing with the kids and other things that

129

make us feel really good. In getting back to doing these things, without focussing too much on the pain having to go away, we make the life circle bigger and pain is taking up less of the space. The pain doesn't necessarily have to go away for us to start living our lives again. Many people find when changing their focus like this, over time, pain may gradually reduce, or it becomes much less of a big deal for them. They are able to cope with the pain because their life is much fuller and more enjoyable.

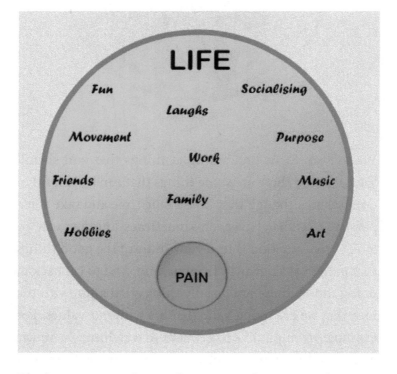

The best way to take on this approach is to use the same

pacing approach as we described earlier for exercise rehabilitation. If you were wanting to start spending some time playing the piano, you might start with just two minutes to begin with, and then build up gradually. If getting out and socialising has been a problem because of extended times needed to sit or stand, choose to catch up for a coffee with a friend and keep the visit short. Start small and build up. It can be helpful to identify some of the areas of your life that you feel pain has really interfered with, work out what "things" you have actually stopped doing because of the pain, and work out ways to start to work towards doing those things. Treating them like rehabilitation goals can be helpful to make them happen – schedule them into your week and do the planning that needs to be done to ensure that they happen.

Stress and pain

Because of those connections between our stress hormones and pain, recognising and reducing stress can be a really big part of getting better. Even just the stress around worrying that you are damaging your tissues or going to make things worse can play into your pain levels. Understanding that pain doesn't mean that tissue damage is occurring can take a big load off your mind and reduce the worry that tends to go hand in hand with pain. Other things that can be helpful to reduce the impact that stress is having on your pain levels might include seeing a psychologist and trying some mindfulness exercises. Psychologists have played a strong and important role in pain management teams for many years. Seeing a psychologist doesn't mean that your pain is not real or is all in your head. It can be really helpful way to look at all the factors in your life that are contributing to your pain. They can also help you to develop strategies to cope, including how you might review your thoughts around pain and your situation to help you place things in a more positive frame. There is very good evidence in the scientific literature to demonstrate that seeing a psychologist and using either cognitive behavioral therapy (CBT) or acceptance and commitment therapy (ACT) approaches significantly improves function, and reduces distress for people in pain. Seeking out someone who works specifically with people in pain or who uses these approaches can be helpful. It can also be good to remember that you may need to find the right person for you, so ask your doctor or other health professionals for recommendations, and be prepared to try another person if you feel they are not a good fit for you.

Mindfulness can be a helpful tool to reduce stress and tension in your body. The easiest way to get started is to use an app on your phone or an internet based program.

Using mindfulness can seem a bit esoteric when pain is affecting a region of your body. It is not designed to take your pain away, but to help the mind be calmer throughout the day. This makes it better able to deal with the ups and downs of the day and ultimately calms a busy mind. Like many of the other active strategies that we use to help a person in pain, it doesn't work to totally take the pain away, but it can be part of the process to getting better. It also takes time for it to start having an effect so patience and persistence is required.

Resources

Below are some good resources that can be really helpful to use to help embrace this bigger picture approach to getting better.

Explain Pain

This book is a great place to start to learn more about pain and how to get better. It is written by David Butler and Lorimer Moseley. You might recognise the name – many of our Pain Heroes found it to be of great benefit. It can be purchased as an e-book, an audiobook or book via the NOI website www.noigroup.com or you could ask if your local library has a copy.

The Protectometor

Going hand in hand with this book is The Protectometor written by the same team. It is a workbook that you can purchase online or as a book and is designed to be worked through to identify the things in life that could be contributing to pain and the areas that can hep a person to get better. It is fabulous and well worth purchasing and is available via the same link as Explain Pain above.

Painful Yarns

A great book by Lorimer Moseley that gives wonderful insight into how different people experience pain. It has some great analogies and stories and is an entertaining read and is also available on the NOI website above.

Recovery Guide

Another resource that I have used with patients and they have found very helpful is the Recovery Guide by Greg Lehman. This extensive resource can be downloaded here. http://www.greglehman.ca/pain-science-work-books/ Greg is an incredibly knowledgeable and experienced clinician and he generously allows this to be freely downloaded with a donation option.

The Pain Toolkit

Pete Moore, whose story featured earlier created this fabulous Pain Toolkit that helps people with self management of persistent pain. www.paintoolkit.org

Why Pelvic Pain Hurts

This is a great resource by experts in their field – Adriaan Louw, Sandra Hilton and Carolyn Vandyken.

A Guide To Better Movement

Todd Hargrove wrote this great guide to movement. He has a great understanding of pain science and how to recover from pain. It is available in a book and e-book.

Mindfulness resources:

Smiling Mind

This is a free resource that has great information and actual mindfulness sessions available via the website and an App that can be downloaded to your phone. It follows a program that takes you through how to do mindfulness meditation. You can also pick and choose the sessions that you enjoy the most. https://www.smilingmind.com.au

Headspace

This is also a great resource that has both an App and information on the website. You can access a free trial period before signing up to relatively inexpensive mindfulness course. https://www.headspace.com

Finding the right practitioner to help the recovery journey can be an important step. It will need to be someone who understands pain science and embraces active approaches over passive approaches. Remember that you might need to try a few practitioners to find the right fit for you.

A pain specialist (medical doctor) can be a good practitioner to have on your team. They can help to guide medication or other interventions if they think they will be helpful, can rule out anything that has been missed and will know good allied health professionals to create a team around you. This team based approach is known to get the best results for people with persistent pain.

SOME HELPFUL SUMMARIES

Pacing

Pacing is an important concept to help you to return to doing the things that you love – things that pain often takes away from us. Understanding this concept is the key to balance improving your function without increasing your pain levels too often.

- **Slowly Slowly.** Our bodies can cope with gradual increases in activity, but they don't like big spikes in activity. Often when we do too much, too soon, we might experience a temporary increase in pain.
- **Plan.** The key to pacing is having a plan to "Pace up" whatever the activity is you would like to do and then to stick to it. One of the key concepts with pacing is that you *stick to the plan* when it comes to increasing activity and *not how you are feeling*. This is because our pain levels don't always give us a really clear indication of where things are at – they

can underestimate how well our tissues are coping, and that can also overestimate if we are experiencing some discomfort.

- **Be Patient.** Often starting low and going slow can be boring and frustrating, especially if we were used to being able to do the activities without a second thought. Sticking to the graded incremental increases in your pacing plan help to prevent the *"Boom and Bust"* that often happens as we try to return to activities.

- **It is Ok to experience some pain.** It doesn't mean you are damaging your tissues. Small increases in your baseline pain levels are ok as you start to move more. Stick to the plan to achieve the activity level that you had planned for that day rather than stopping or reducing the activity because of transient pain. If you experience unmanageable pain during the activity then you should stop.

- **Exposure and Resilience.** When we start increasing our activity levels slowly, it helps the tissues to adapt at a level that they can cope with. This slow exposure helps make the tissues gradually more resilient and shows you that you have the capacity to improve.

- **You can "Pace Up" anything!** If there is something that you would like to start doing again, use the pacing principles. You can try it for: walking, sitting, driving, cooking, gardening, work related activities.

Start really low and try to make sure that you have success at each increment

- **Fatigue.** Pacing works really well to combat fatigue. You use exactly the same ideas to increase your tolerance to fatigue as you would to general activities.
- **Use numbers.** To set your pacing plan, use tangible, measurable increments to increase your activities. You might set a timer, count numbers or repetitions, measure your heart rate and set a target for it or count your daily steps with a pedometer. As long as you use the same system it doesn't really matter. Its important to stop when the plan says to stop, not to decide based on how you are feeling.
- **If you flare up – don't freak out!** Finding the level at which you can stay comfortably under that flare up threshold, but work hard enough to make change is tricky! It requires patience and persistence. Sometimes you might hit that threshold in a pacing approach. *Don't panic!* It will pass, and the positive is that you know where that threshold is and can work just under it.

Managing Flare Ups

- **If you flare up – don't freak out!** It is normal and even somewhat expected to feel times of increased pain when you have persistent pain. This is especially the case if you are starting to increase your levels of activity. Know that it will pass and that you haven't done damage to your tissues.

- **Arm yourself.** Develop a basket of tricks to help deal with temporary increases in pain as they pass and the unhelpful thoughts that often accompany this. These might include using heat or ice, gentle stretching or exercises, relaxation techniques, hot showers or self massage. Some people can find the use of a TENS machine to be useful at these times. Its also important to have discussed medication for pain increases with your doctor before it happens. Review your thoughts to ensure they are empowering you and to ensure that these are not contributing to the pain and suffering you are experiencing during the flare up. Having a plan and knowing what to do can take the stress out of flare ups and make you feel more in control.

- **Do Something.** The temptation when experiencing high levels of pain is just to do nothing. Whilst it might make sense intuitively, we know that this leads to further deconditioning which can lower your threshold to experience more pain. Keep doing something during times of increased pain, even if it is just a fraction of what you might normally do and try to make it something that you enjoy or will help you overall. Know that you are not damaging your tissues.

- **Avoid overdoing it.** Knowing what triggers a flare

up for you can be a helpful way to avoid frequently having temporary increases in pain. If you have pain, try to review what you have done in the recent past that might have brought it on. If you can identify what might have contributed, don't avoid doing that thing in the future, just be sure to use Pacing principles when you go back to it. Sometimes there may not be a trigger for your flare up that you can identify. Thats ok too! When our nervous systems are very sensitive, as they are in persistent pain, sometimes even stress can increase our pain.

- **Get back on track.** As soon as your pain settles down to levels prior to the flare up, resume your activities. Frequent flare ups are a quick way to hijack a good rehabilitation plan so its important to resume your activities and keep moving onwards and upwards.

ABOUT THE AUTHOR

Alison Sim is a clinician who has been working especially with persistent pain patients for many years. She also has a keen interest in educating health professionals about the latest science surrounding pain.

Alison qualified as an osteopath in 2001. She has a Masters of Science in Medicine in Pain Management from Sydney University Medical School and Royal North Shore Pain Management Research Institute. She has lectured at Australian Catholic University, Victoria University, RMIT and George Fox University in a variety of science and clinical subjects. She has also worked as part of the teaching team at Deakin University Medical School and is currently based in Melbourne, Australia.

She runs workshops and lectures for clinicians on topics related to pain both face to face and online.

She has a blog and other resources at www.beyondmechanicalpain.com